# PATHS TO THE ALEXANDER TECHNIQUE

Paths to the Alexander Technique
First published in 2015 by HITE

Copyright © 2015 The F. Matthias Alexander Trust
All rights reserved. No part of this publication may be reproduced, stored in a retrieval system or transmitted in any form or by any means, electronic, mechanical, photocopying, recording or otherwise, without the prior written permission of the publisher.

A CIP catalogue for this book is available from the British Library.

Cover image and design: N Thapen

Printed and bound in UK by Imprint Digital

ISBN: 9780956899767

# Contents

| | |
|---|---|
| Acknowledgements | i |
| **Prologue** | **iii** |
| **First Encounters with the Alexander Technique** | **1** |
| 'Not Doing' in Daily Life - *Nick Branch* | 5 |
| Facing Each Day in My Life - *Jacqui Hinton* | 7 |
| Musician and Composer - *Chris Cousin* | 10 |
| British Soldier, Australian Alexander Technique Teacher - *Mike McGurgan* | 12 |
| Conference Interpreter, Alexander Technique Teacher, Mother - *Anna Cooper* | 16 |
| Taking Control of a Body and a Life - *Peter Ribeaux* | 20 |
| **Recognition of the Force of Habit** | **23** |
| The Fundamental Core of My Existence - *Clarissa Palmer* | 25 |
| My Experience of the Alexander Technique as a Musician - *Teresa Turner* | 30 |
| The Experience of an 'Older Person' - *Dorothy Walker* | 34 |
| Council Worker, Speech Therapist - *Sean Richardson* | 38 |
| Why I Study the Alexander Technique - *Dorothy Jerrome* | 42 |
| Reflections - *Janette Griffin* | 45 |
| The Long Road to the Carriage-Driving Trials Championship - *Karen Scott-Barrett* | 49 |
| Using the Alexander Technique in Liturgy and Teaching - *Father Alcuin Schachenmayr* | 52 |
| **Inhibition** | **55** |
| The Twelve Pound Tale - *Helen May* | 57 |
| My Journey to the Alexander Technique, Surgery and Beyond - *Mary Rawson* | 63 |
| The Way Back from Losing a Voice and a Career - *Keith Hawkins* | 69 |
| The Freedom to Ascend - *Jennet Blake* | 71 |
| Never Too Old to Start - *Thomas Newton* | 72 |
| The Emerging Self - *Jane Evans* | 78 |

| | |
|---|---:|
| **Unreliable Sensory Appreciation** | **87** |
| Forward and Up at Seventy-Five - *Roey Burden* | 89 |
| Noticing Myself - *Christine Green* | 95 |
| Getting the Horse to Move - *Anonymous* | 98 |
| Twisting to the Right While Leaning to the Left<br>- *Richard Brennan* | 100 |
| Small Surprises When You Don't Expect Them<br>- *Anne Landa* | 105 |
| Working Through the Contractions - *Katie Dixon* | 110 |
| The Tree Branch - *Anonymous* | 112 |
| Discovering the Liberated Breath - *Simon Spire* | 116 |
| **Sending Directions** | **127** |
| Massage Therapy, Kick Boxing and Pole Dancing<br>- *Julia Buccetti* | 129 |
| 'No' is Not a Negative - *Rosemary Nott* | 132 |
| Gentle but Effective - *Melody Hirst* | 140 |
| Memories in the Making - *Amie Shorey* | 143 |
| The Beagler - *Anonymous* | 147 |
| **The Primary Control of the Use of the Self** | **149** |
| The Wheel Comes Full Circle - *Veronica Pollard* | 151 |
| The Real Deal - *David Green* | 153 |
| Leaving the Feet Behind - *Kerry Downes* | 164 |
| The Alexander Technique - My Personal Story<br>- *Geraldeen Fitzgerald* | 168 |
| A Mindfulness Trail Through the Forest - *Cherry Collins* | 172 |
| Round and Round the Garden: A Spiral Learning Journey<br>- *Carolyn Nicholls* | 178 |
| Destiny Shapes Our Ends - *Ann Smith* | 183 |
| **Epilogue** | **191** |
| **Glossary** | **195** |
| **Bibliography** | **201** |

# Acknowledgements

Credit for the idea for this book goes to Jean Clark, Di Maclellan and Mary Walker, and to The F. Matthias Alexander Trust for supporting and financing its production. Thanks are also due to the Society of Teachers of the Alexander Technique (STAT), who promoted and supported the idea in Statnews, and to the STAT office staff for their generous help.

A big thank you to Claire de Obaldia for writing the Prologue and Epilogue and contributing to the introductions, and to Peter Ribeaux for helping collate and organise the stories and the section introductions. Thanks also to Emily Bates for proofreading the manuscript.

Finally, The F. Matthias Alexander Trust would like to express a huge thank you to all of the authors who have shared their stories with us. They have had to wait a long time to see them in print and we hope they feel, as we do, the value of bringing the Alexander Technique to a wider audience.

# Prologue

The men and women who have agreed to share their stories with us came across the work of F.M. Alexander because they felt they were not functioning to the best of their capacities. The trigger was a crisis or a problem they needed to solve with varying degrees of urgency: a life-changing trauma, such as a severe and debilitating pain after a serious accident; a condition or chronic disorder – perhaps congenital, perhaps resulting from an illness or, in the case of back pain, from an unfortunate movement – which suddenly became worse. Less dramatically, it might have been a block of some kind, or a sense of a 'lifestyle becoming more and more restricted', as Melody Hirst puts it. Or they felt that they were not able to tap into their potential properly, and life was passing them by.

Often the aim is to find a rapid and effective solution, and the Alexander Technique tends to be the last resort, after a number of other, more obvious remedies (including various forms of alternative therapy) have been tried to no avail. Eventually – by hearsay, through a GP, a friend, an article in a magazine, a television interview, something heard on the radio, a poster, a leaflet, an adult education class, by chancing upon one of Alexander's books, or by being offered a first lesson as a birthday present – our storytellers, randomly and often sceptically, turn to the Alexander Technique. They feel they have 'nothing more to lose', and 'the risks attached to trying out the Technique are so low – no medicaments, no surgery – and moderate costs', as the author of The Beagler's story says. They discover that the Technique is gentle and non-intrusive.

It is so non-intrusive, in fact, that in the Alexander lesson there will probably be no question of treating the specific complaint at all. Rather than concerning themselves with it the teacher usually chooses to attend to how their new pupil coordinates mind and body, or how they 'use' themselves in typical, everyday situations.

Rosemary Nott's experience is quite typical in this regard: 'After a certain number of lessons, I pursued again the question of "Would this help my feet as well as my back?"… "I don't see why not," said my teacher. No further elucidation, no further discussion about my feet – she didn't even look at them... So I began to forget about the feet and they were rarely mentioned again.'

Having chanced upon the Alexander Technique indirectly, not to say inadvertently, for a condition which is also going to be tackled indirectly, what a surprise when something *does* happen! When (or, you might argue, because) nothing much seems to be happening in the expected sense, a change takes place. The condition which they have been invited to approach indirectly has become manageable, or has mysteriously disappeared.

From overcoming an initial limitation, our narrators find they can not only make the most of the condition they live with, but push their limits and discover abilities, dispositions, skills which they never thought they had, or which they had simply been afraid to try out. The improvement of a predominantly physical condition may open up a world of unexpected physical possibilities and conversely, sorting out an apparently more 'mental' problem may unexpectedly lift other psychological blocks, or simply broaden the mental repertoire.

In the last resort it seems there is nothing the Alexander Technique cannot be successfully applied to: our bike-rider (Veronica Pollard) gets gradually better at riding her bike, but also gets better at 'just about everything else'; our conference interpreter emphasises the 'invaluable' benefits of 'using the Technique in the high-pressure environment of conference interpreting', but also remarks that it is 'just as useful in dealing with one's child's headmistress, walking the Surrey hills, catching a ball … or coping with tax return[s]'; Dorothy Jerrome

*Prologue*

finds the Technique in a roundabout way when initially 'searching for an effective therapy' for her husband and comes to value the AT for 'physical, emotional, aesthetic, philosophical, [and] intellectual reasons'.

It is this wonder and joy that, in seeking relief for a specific complaint or condition, or to improve a specific skill, should have taken them on the fascinating journey of self-discovery, from life enhancing to life changing, that our narrators want to share with us. Their stories are unique, and yet, to echo the wish expressed by Cherry Collins at the beginning of her own story, 'may aspects of these stories speak to you in whatever form is helpful to you now'.

*Claire de Obaldia*

# First Encounters with the Alexander Technique

Have you ever felt the need to find a way to manage back pain, to play your instrument better, to increase your self confidence, to recover faster from a serious accident, to take control of certain aspects of your life, or to ease some of the difficulties of old age?

Can it be that there is a skill that can be learned which provides a 'yes' answer to all of these? According to the authors of the stories in this book, the answer is, there is.

This book had its origin in a request for people who had had lessons in the Alexander Technique to write down their stories. Our thanks go to those who responded. The book offers a collection of people's experiences in relation to life events which were, for them, the occasion for rehabilitation and growth. It also serves as an indirect introduction to the Alexander Technique.

There were many ways that these stories could have been selected and ordered. In the end we opted to stay as close to Alexander as possible and use five of his concepts for the purpose, choosing those which, according to Macdonald (1989), taken together distinguish the Alexander Technique from other disciplines (*The Alexander Technique as I See It*, p. 86).

The concepts are: *the recognition of the force of habit, inhibition and non-doing, unreliable sensory appreciation, sending directions* and *the primary control of the use of the self*. At the beginning of each section, and in this introduction, for the benefit of those not familiar with the

Alexander Technique, there is a short description of the concept as it is illustrated in the stories.

The first group of stories has been chosen to give a flavour of the Technique as a whole, the stories each beginning as they do with the words, 'I first heard of the Alexander Technique' or a very similar phrase, and covering as they do more than one concept. The remaining sections cover the five concepts.

*Recognition of the Force of Habit*
Man is beset by his own habits. Not that habits are a bad thing. We could not live without them. We have a limited capacity for processing information. Thus, making regularly repeated activities habitual and (to a degree) unconscious allows us to function in the present. The way we walk is habitual: we do not often think about the process of walking while talking to a companion (or, increasingly, on the mobile phone) as we carry on our daily life. And so on…

However, some habits are harmful: the way we bend may cause us pain; the way we play the violin may prevent us from reaching our potential as a violinist. The Alexander Technique is a means of accessing dysfunctional habits and consciously choosing to replace them with better ones. It is a means of exercising choice in the way we respond to the stimuli of life.

This 'means whereby' we access and change habits is described by the four remaining concepts of inhibition, giving directions, unreliable sensory appreciation, and the primary control of the use of the self, ideas which interlock to form the Alexander Technique.

*Inhibition*
Firstly, in order to give ourselves choice, we need to prevent or inhibit our immediate reaction to initiate a habit.

This starts with inhibiting any psycho-physical distortions (e.g. tensions) which are about to interfere with our response. Inhibition is a two-stage process which involves firstly pausing before reacting and then preventing the distortion which is about to intervene.

## Sending Directions

Once this inhibition has taken place, we are in a position to work out a means of reacting differently. To do this we need to give our self two sets of guiding instructions or orders. One set establishes a coordinated state of the organism and the other gives consent to a chosen response. This course of action is not without its difficulties; the most important is due to our unreliable sensory appreciation.

## Unreliable Sensory Appreciation

This concept means exactly what it seems to, namely, that our feelings (in particular our bodily sensations) may not be reliable. In practical terms our familiar old habits are likely to feel comfortable (even if they are causing pain or other disturbance). Any new kind of response may feel uncomfortable, awkward or even painful. This is not a defect in the organism but an adaptive characteristic. Our limited capacity for processing information means that as we learn to walk as toddlers, for example, we take into account all sorts of sensations. But once the skill is acquired, we do not pay attention to these sensations. The manner of standing and walking becomes habitual and unconscious. This enables other activities to occupy our attention.

If, however, we want to change our manner of walking – for example, in order to prevent a backache – any change is likely to feel initially uncomfortable, awkward or stilted.

## The Primary Control of the Use of the Self

This is the unifying feature in the process of practising the Alexander Technique. In fact, there are two concepts here: firstly, primary control and secondly, the use of the self.

The term *primary control* refers to both an anatomical entity and a mental activity, that is, both an underlying physiological mechanism and the means of controlling it.

> *I wish to make it clear that when I employ the word 'use', it is not in that limited sense of the use of any specific part, as, for instance, when we speak of the use of an arm or the use of a leg, but in a much wider and more comprehensive sense applying to*

> *the working of the organism in general. For I recognize that the use of any specific part such as the arm or leg involves of necessity bringing into action the different psycho-physical mechanisms of the organism, this concerted activity bringing about the use of the specific part. (The Use of the Self, 1932, p. 22n).*

To summarise, practising the Alexander Technique consists in preventing distortions in the use of ourselves in our everyday activities by means of the primary control of that use. Any changes we make by the processes of inhibition and direction may well feel unfamiliar and strange – even wrong, initially. We can check their appropriateness by observing ourselves (as Alexander did with mirrors) or by having others observe us (a teacher, for example).

Each of these concepts will be further explored at the beginning of each section. The terms, used in Alexander's sense, differ subtly from their dictionary definitions; in keeping with their holistic nature, the concepts are not discrete, but merge into each other as an organic whole. Each section of the book is preceded by one or more quotations selected from Alexander's writings. Full details of the publications are given in the Bibliography. The Glossary may be useful for some of the specialised terminology used by some of the authors.

I hope readers will enjoy this selection of real life stories and that it will enrich their understanding of the Alexander Technique.

*Peter Ribeaux*

# 'Not Doing' in Daily Life
## Nick Branch

I first heard of the Alexander Technique from a friend, who described it as a 'cure for bad posture' after hearing me complaining of the lower-back pain which plagued me for several years in my late teens and early twenties. In fact, it was not just sporadic lower-back pain I suffered with, but neck pain, stiff shoulders, a bad knee, a sore hip – the list went on.

I wasn't in bad shape, although my injuries frequently prevented regular exercise. Because I considered myself fit and healthy, these unexplained setbacks were all the more exasperating.

The first thing that struck me about the Alexander Technique, in contrast to other methods for back pain I had tried, was that it is not described as a 'treatment'. Whilst my physical condition and history were recorded, the Technique is not targeted at curing specific ailments. My teacher described herself first and foremost as a 'teacher', and our weekly thirty minute sessions were described as 'lessons'.

This did not make a great deal of sense to begin with, and the lessons themselves seemed somewhat abstract. We looked at standing up and sitting down, and associated movements. We looked at the 'directions' which form the basis of the Technique. Counter-intuitively, we spent a good deal of time focusing on 'not doing'. When learning something new, I expected there to be a skill or an action to grasp and perfect, but the Alexander Technique is firstly about 'not doing'. In fact, learning not to do, in spite of burning compulsion – to intervene, to act, to move, to do – is something which can be applied successfully in many other situations in daily life.

My natural scepticism initially told me that these alien concepts might not be worth the time of day and expense. And yet there was something in those early sessions. It was a step into the unknown, and I felt like progress was being made. That many other people before me had had faith in the Technique was a comfort, and that many of these were actors, musicians, performers of the very highest order gave further credibility.

One of the biggest hurdles for me was reconciling my investment of time and money not only with myself but with others interested in what I was doing. It is a difficult concept to explain, but results speak for themselves, and within a few months the random back pain had vanished. I was also noticing benefits I hadn't expected. My reactions were sharper; I felt more confident, more focused. I was not consciously doing anything different, and yet I felt quite different. Whilst practising standing up and sitting down felt at certain times somewhat ridiculous, when I thought about it, I spend most of my life sat on chairs, standing, walking, lying down. To learn to do these things better was to improve my performance in some of the activities I do the most, and yet think about the least.

As my confidence grew, I was able to apply the principles of the Technique to other activities in my life, including running, swimming and cycling. Mastering better body use facilitates improved performance, and I became more competent in all these pursuits. I ran half marathons with no lasting knee problems. I cycled a thousand miles in twelve days for charity, without issues. I have become a far better swimmer than I ever was before, and my tennis (previously all forehand and very little else) has developed considerably.

I have now been seeing my teacher for three years, for much of this time with a weekly lesson, but latterly with a fortnightly 45-minute session. With hindsight and experience, weekly lessons helped enforce the new thought patterns. In our lessons we have looked at many different areas of movement, breathing, posture and balance. I look forward to bringing observations on my own use and issues with my learning to someone with so much knowledge, not only of the Technique but of wider anatomy.

As I move to a new phase in my own life, I remain confident that the Alexander Technique will continue to play a part. Only once you have started to learn do you realise how vast the subject of body use is, and how feasibly limitless are the improvements that can be made.

# Facing Each Day in My Life
## Jacqui Hinton

The first time I encountered the Alexander Technique was when staying on business in a small village just outside Abingdon in Oxfordshire, around 2007. The setting was stunning: not the usual bed-and-breakfast type of property; it was a lovingly restored manor house. The landlady was able to offer guests Alexander Technique lessons. At the time I thought it was well worth bearing in mind for the next visit, which sadly never took place.

In May 2010, I remembered about my brief brush with the Alexander Technique teacher in Oxfordshire, and found the information I had got at the time. Thanks to the Internet, typing 'Alexander Technique in the Midlands' brought about the discovery of a website with a directory of Alexander teachers. In visiting the teachers' websites, I found one Midlands-based teacher I was drawn to, a very important part of any therapy, I feel.

Waiting to receive that first response call to my telephone message, I remember, felt different from most. It's hard to describe, but today, ten months on from calling this lady, I can only look forwards to facing each day in my life, which at the time was so hard to imagine ever doing again. On the second day of 2009 my world as I had known it stopped turning: I lost my adoptive mother that day to a series of strokes. This scenario was in fact to be the first of three. I was told a month later the results of an MRI scan requested by my GP and backed up by a letter of concern from my osteopath.

The last fourteen months of the decline in my elderly mother saw my own heath disappearing: the loss of reflex feeling in the whole of the right side of my body, and very little on the left, had to be addressed. The way forward recommended by the medical profession was to get an MRI scan first; the results came one month after losing my mother. I was shown one slipped disc in the lower back, and another one which had started to move.

Working very successfully for myself with a transport training business, teaching men and women all over the UK from every walk of life to drive all sizes and types of trucks, was to be no more after being given the MRI scan results. Twenty-four years of pioneering as a female truck-driving instructor and breaking down the barriers in more ways than one – also being from an ethnic minority, British-born and educated privately in the male-orientated transport industry – ended. Going against medical advice, due to losing my mother, I continued to train drivers and eleven months down the line, the business was over, not just because of my medical condition, but also because of the economic decline in the country.

I started the Alexander Technique in May and ten months on, with lessons weekly, most of the time I have become confident and happy to rebuild life slowly and in a still manner; I had never experienced this prior to taking Alexander Technique lessons.

I owe so much to my AT teacher. A unique bond has formed over the ten months I have known her, and because the lessons are one-to-one and the setting being in a comfortable private home, it's just right for me.

The changes were made over a relatively short period of time, not quite forty lessons, I think at this point and in my case, forty-five minutes a week. The powers of this work are inexhaustible. Full belief and confidence in the world of the Alexander work and your teacher must be present in every sense of the word. Self-investment in re-education for the use of your own body, mind and spirit coordinated to function as one, that's how I have now come to understand and experience the Alexander Technique.

The experience of having your body and mind looked at and examined in a whole new way by a stranger in their own home feels odd at first, it really does. The way I overcame my concerns and worries, if you like, of the work was to research the Alexander Technique, starting with the gentleman Mr F.M. Alexander's life and his fascinating discovery, to a point where I sometimes feel I have met this remarkable man.

The information from the Internet, in the form of websites and watching YouTube, not to mention reading numerous books, all make this globally practised Technique clearer by the minute.

All that remains to be said is 'thanks' to my teacher, who is worth her weight in gold. My life has been changed for good. If it's meant, maybe one day I will become a teacher myself, who knows?

## Musician and Composer
### Chris Cousin

I am a musician and composer in my early forties. By the time I reached my early thirties, I had had three serious whiplash injuries in the previous twenty years, resulting in pain all over my back and constant headaches. I had been doing Tai Chi for something like eight or nine years and was considered to be a senior student who knew what he was doing. But Tai Chi was aggravating the problem in my back, so, reluctantly, I had to let go of that and find something else. I started yoga and the Alexander Technique at the same time.

The Tai Chi teacher had told me about the Alexander Technique in the past and I had read *The Use of the Self*, but then I met someone who had some kind of congenital problem with her spine and lots of back problems. She had gone down the medical route and said that the Alexander Technique had helped her enormously, and that was what made me think I'd go and have a lesson.

The effects have been that I rarely have headaches, and I'd say I get twenty percent of the back problems that I had then. I did yoga classes for about a year, and I really enjoyed it and got a lot out of it because I could do it, but after a year of that I realised that my back hurt just as much as it did at the beginning.

After about a year or so, I heard of a friend who had been for a yoga therapy in London after pregnancy and did one-to-one sessions, so then I pursued that route. I had also read Desikachar's *Heart of Yoga*. It seemed to be very intelligent, and a very balanced view, but there were also some things that attracted me. For instance, he was talking about how to measure one's progress in yoga, saying that it's not about how you can stand on your head or how far you can stretch. It is in one's relationships with other people that you measure your progress. Reflecting on that and the attitude of the teacher, I started to think that there was something missing. Anyway, I went for one-to-one lessons with the teacher who gave me a really simple practice, nothing fancy whatsoever, for ten to fifteen minutes, and I would always use the Alexander Technique to do the yoga. It is difficult to separate the benefits of the Alexander Technique and yoga if you do both at the same time.

After I'd had maybe ten or twenty Alexander Technique lessons I could say there was an improvement in my back. Finally, I was able to do something to get some improvement. Then, I guess it was probably four or five years after going to see the second yoga teacher, she invited me on a course with her teacher. He basically works in such a similar way to the Alexander Technique, but one of his strong teaching points is how you focus the mind while practising the posture, and there was an enormous similarity between his concepts and the Technique. Then I just pursued that. I have pursued working with him in the last four or five years or so, as well as pursuing the Technique. I would say I probably get equal benefit from each. He is a remarkable man. He can bring you to the same place, if you want to call it that, the same experience in a similar way (without having to touch you) as a really good Alexander teacher.

I still go and see a chiropractor regularly. I still get aches in my back, my neck still gets locked up.

Through the Technique, I've realised that there are things I do that aggravate those whiplash injuries. But the other side to it is my attitude to life. I find that I'm calmer, have a clearer head. I'm able to concentrate in a less restrictive way. I find that I enjoy things more, I enjoy my life much more. I have more pleasure. Everything in life is much richer, which means that the difficult things in life are much more vivid. I experience the negative emotions much more fully than I did, but I am able to just let them pass quicker than they did; so the difficult things in life are just a little bit less difficult. The pleasurable things in life are a little bit more pleasurable. This is after something like one hundred lessons over a period of ten years; so it's no magic bullet. I had fifty-five lessons with my local teacher. I must have had twenty-five to thirty days in Alexander teacher-training schools; so I'm a bit of an Alexander groupie!

# British Soldier, Australian Alexander Technique Teacher
Mike McGurgan

I was serving as a warrant officer in an elite corps on peace-keeping duties in Northern Ireland during the 1970s when one of my men began behaving oddly. When he was transferred out, having been diagnosed with what is now called PTSD (post-traumatic stress disorder), I began researching. I started reading up on the subject. One book had a reference to the Alexander Technique, and that began the quest. But it was eleven years before I was able to experience a lesson, when an advert appeared in a local newspaper on the Isle of Man. By this time I had completed my pensionable engagement and retired from military life. The advert said 'Alexander Technique' and gave a telephone number. They were the only words I saw on the page! The teacher was on the Island for only ten days so I booked five lessons on the spur of the moment – it just felt right!

Following the directions I was given, I parked and walked toward the main road, not realising that I had parked on the wrong side of it. Not finding the cottage, I asked a passing young lady, 'Could you tell me the way to Rose Cottage, please?' She replied, 'You must be Mike!'

Seeing the look of incredulity on my face, she replied, 'I teach the Alexander Technique. I'm staying at Rose Cottage and my next client – in ten minutes time – is Mike!'

'Bloody Hell!' I said, 'what a technique!'

So as we walked toward the cottage we just kept bursting out laughing and by the time we reached it, it was as if we'd known each other all our lives.

I don't remember much about the first lesson, except that there was some chair work and a table turn, and a cup of tea. But when I walked back to my car it was as if all the 'treacle' had dissolved, (that's the only way I can describe it). It was as if, previous to the lesson, my movements had been restricted like I was wading through treacle.

Also, having suffered from constipation since childhood, it was wonderful, that evening to have a 'normal' bowel movement.

The next four lessons passed all too quickly, and then there was a three-month wait until the teacher returned to the Island. This had occurred four more times, when one day she said, 'Have you thought about training to teach the Technique?'

I said, 'I couldn't do what you do.' And she said, 'Oh yes, you could, think about it'.

Three months later, when she returned and put her hands on my shoulders, I was sitting in a chair, she exclaimed 'Good God! What have you been doing to yourself?' I said that I'd been thinking about what had been said previously and that there were too many problems in the way.

Her reply was, 'Well, who is making the problems? Why don't you take a step at a time and just see what happens!'

So next the morning, early, before breakfast, I looked through the information that I had, and four training schools leapt out at me. After writing letters, I received invitations from them to call. So I worked out an itinerary.

After visiting the schools and being almost overwhelmed with friendliness and the attention I received, and the concerns for my welfare, I reluctantly returned to the Isle of Man. Within five months I had sold my business, separated from my then-wife of twenty years and relocated to Exeter, within easy commuting distance of the Alexander Technique school that I had chosen to attend.

The three-year training course I found amazing, with students aged from twenty-five to sixty-eight years, and occupations ranging from a physiotherapist with a practice near Harley Street, to a plasterer, an actor, a document translator, a Danish girl (whose training and expenses were paid for by the Danish government!) and a German theatre manager, actor and acrobat, who was living and working in Sweden. Then there was me, with my military posture that took eighteen months to even begin to free up, so that I could breathe with ease, and in the process release twenty-two years or more of emotional holding, and so come to terms with my own PTSD. The course was a rollercoaster, with periods of intense calm and beauty and extreme emotion, which passed all too quickly.

On graduating in July 1996, I returned to the Isle of Man and, with the help of friends, was accommodated and set up in practice, firstly in a 'front room' in a private house, and eventually in purpose-built premises co-located with a doctor in private practice, with a receptionist and 'brass plate' on the door!

In 2000, I met Amanda, when she brought her fifteen year-old daughter for a lesson. She was a single mother with three teenagers. Ever up for a challenge, I courted her for a year before we married in September, 2001. Grace was born December, 2002. One year later we moved off the Island, as it had become a 'tax haven', and tried living in Plymouth, England; then moved to Kerala, South India for a year, teaching in a school (attached to an ashram) and giving private lessons. It was during this year that we found Australia. To avoid 'the Wet' in India and to visit Amanda's relations, we holidayed in Australia and fell in love with the people, the country and the culture.

Back in India, we visited a neighbour who had originally come from Melbourne. She was married to an Ayurvedic doctor and had recently been appointed as an Australian immigration agent. We accepted her offer to begin the process of applying for a visa. We were her first clients. Three years later, we arrived in Tamworth, New South Wales! Amanda applied to an agency in Helsinki for an RN post the same day that Tamworth Rural Referral Hospital applied for an RN! The happy coincidences continued. Three days after arriving, Amanda was trying out a second-hand car when I noticed the number plate had her initials on it! It was meant to be.

*First Encounters with the Alexander Technique*

The same day, we were called in to the estate agent's office to discuss a house that we had put an offer on, and found that there was an option to rent the property while we were waiting for 'foreign investment approval', which took about eight weeks. We were in our own little home within three weeks of setting foot in Australia!

I am not only a member of AUSTAT, but have been appointed to the Training Course Standing Committee as well as running a growing private practice. Amanda, visa requirements fulfilled, now works part-time. Grace has represented her school in swimming and athletics, and is growing into a 'typical Aussie'. Life is good!

## Conference Interpreter, Alexander Technique Teacher, Mother
Anna Cooper

I first encountered the Alexander Technique in 1972. Training to be a conference interpreter in London, I was nervous of microphones and the prospect of speaking to hundreds of people. And I was not confident with my unsophisticated, lower-middle-class accent – it needed to be improved, more middle class. A fellow trainee was seeing Michael McCallion, a voice coach from RADA, and thought he might be able to help.

'You'll have to work on your accent by yourself, darling,' said Michael. 'As to feeling confident on mike, have you heard of the Alexander Technique?'

Several years and many Alexander lessons later I'd become rather entranced by the changes the Technique had made. I was more confident, had been working all over the continent for the EU, had met the man I would marry and was living in Britain again. During a lesson, my teacher mentioned she had seen my name on the waiting list (seven years long!) to train as an Alexander teacher. I was startled. I had not applied, and had no idea how my name had got on to the list. It seemed unfair to keep it there and I asked for it to be removed. That set me thinking. Wouldn't this be a fascinating new departure and a way of not having to travel in order to work? Miraculously, my name was reinstated. I began to train in 1978.

With an address in London, I was awarded a study grant from the Inner London Education Authority – now, sadly, a faded piece of history – and spent three and a half years training in the Alexander Technique. I embarked on the training with uncertain expectations and a concealed dose of scepticism. This was fuelled on my first morning when a senior teacher lying in semi-supine on a nearby table startled me by releasing tension in a disturbing series of menacing growls. I forbore to 'work on myself', deciding I would challenge the Alexander Technique to prove itself first. It took two years before I realised it had.

*First Encounters with the Alexander Technique*

By the time this insight crystallised, I was about to give birth to my first child – pregnancy being an ideal 'app', in contemporary terms, of the Alexander Technique. I had no back pain during this, or my second, pregnancy. Because of motherhood, though, I had to take a term off after my seventh term, then continue training part-time for three further terms.

During the early part of the training course I took up running, taught by Paul Collins in line with Alexander's principles. I ran in a few weekend workshops, following Paul's recommendation to run towards the front of the feet, a principle I have applied ever since. Did we need Daniel Lieberman, a Harvard professor of Human Evolutionary Biology, to tell us that humans were designed to do this? Modern running shoes make it difficult, and commercial gimmickry has given us gel, air, bubbles and so on to cushion the impact on the heel. But who needs them if the shoes are flexible enough for us to land towards the front of the foot as we lengthen the torso and free the neck (when we remember)?

With a young family, I did little teaching and had little contact with colleagues for several years, suppressing an uneasy feeling that my work, both on pupils and on myself, was inferior. During this time I did manage to take lessons from Peggy Williams, Marjorie Barlow, Margaret Goldie, Eric de Peyer and – my favourite – John Skinner, all of whom had worked with Alexander. I found that each had a 'hallmark'. With Marjorie I learned the importance of being realistic with language and concepts; with Margaret I felt I understood more about freeing the neck and not doing; with Eric I learned to be experimental and unafraid; and John Skinner taught me to laugh at the Alexander Technique while taking it very seriously. I always felt I was levitating as I left him, and used it to float up a nearby footbridge. We shared a distaste for idolatry, and felt that one can learn useful tools from many teachers.

Once I could expand my work I found that these years had, in fact, enriched my teaching. I was thrilled when I found myself asking a pupil whether she had ever worn a surgical corset around the lower half of her back and being told that my supposition was correct. It has also been deeply satisfying to be able to help sufferers from chronic disorders such as Parkinson's, Charcot-Marie-Tooth disorder or osteogenesis imperfecta to manage their condition.

Some years ago I trained as a mediator in community disputes. Now there's an opportunity to inhibit! Distaste, irritation, horror, judgementalism are inhibited and then processed constructively for the benefit of the participants in the mediation process. A brilliant training for life, too!

I did not give up occasional interpreting in Brussels, Luxembourg, Strasbourg and so on, but interpreting had to fit around teaching the Alexander Technique, not the other way round. It's a huge privilege to work where you want, when you want and for what you think you are worth. And also to do work you enjoy, and for which your clients regularly express appreciation. It does, though, imply that you have another source of income to pay the bills. It is up to each one of us to spread the word, so that this will gradually change. For over thirty years I have never missed an opportunity of explaining what I do and spreading understanding – no mean challenge!

A perk of the job is the things you learn from the people you teach. Teaching the AT has given me insights into shooting, playing the cello, writing novels, accident and emergency departments, financial planning, silk printing, educational publishing, opera singing, rugby football, garden maintenance, television production, getting old and being a teenager (teenagers are often very receptive to the Alexander Technique).

In my own life, using the Technique in the high-pressure environment of conference interpreting was invaluable to me but it is just as useful in dealing with one's child's headmistress, walking the Surrey hills, catching a ball (which I could never do before) or coping with a tax return. I have even learned to enjoy public speaking, which used to terrify me. These days, when so many of us spend hours at computers, the Technique is a front-line resource in applied ergonomics. In fact, to judge by comments from my clients, this is an area where we teachers have a critical contribution to make.

Speaking several languages, I have brought the Technique to people in France, Belgium, Austria, Switzerland and Germany, mainly friends. It is rewarding when you see people after some years and they report how helpful the semi-supine has been: '..some corner of a foreign field... shaped, made aware...' (with apologies to Rupert Brooke)!

Is there still such a thing as the Alexander Technique? Apart from the core principles, teachers evolve their own tricks creatively and empirically. It has been said that teachers are teaching their own system, based on the Alexander Technique. I believe Alexander would be pleased with this. In *The Use of the Self* he stresses that the results 'can safely be left to take their own form', and science, quoting Dewey, 'is not something finished, absolute in itself'.

The Alexander Technique still has a long way to go in order to reach the wider public and medics. It is gratifying to receive occasional referrals from osteopaths, chiropractors, neurosurgeons or rheumatologists, yet GPs mostly seem to have neither the time nor the motivation to find out about it. Hopefully further research studies will change all that. But the situation today is a far cry from when I started, innocently placing an advertisement for the Technique in a local paper. I was deluged for the next few weeks with telephone calls from gentlemen requiring services which I did not provide!

As my bones get older and my components regularly remind me of the passing years, I am becoming incentivised to apply the Technique more often to avoid pointless visits to doctors' surgeries. No one else is responsible for my biomechanics, though it would sometimes be good to blame someone!

As a professional communicator, when teaching the Technique I have always striven to use plain English to impart the Alexander principles. Language must move with the times; the challenge is to say and do whatever it takes to get the ideas across to each individual learner or organisation. I've always disliked the word 'pupil', sharing John Skinner's view that it sounds patronising. I don't mind being regarded as a therapist. Clients will quickly find that part of the job is theirs, even as I relieve them of their money. Teaching is wonderful when people enjoy learning.

## Taking Control of a Body and a Life
Peter Ribeaux

At the age of nineteen I walked off the squash court one day with a mild lower-back pain. Within a week I was bent over forward like those signs used to indicate the proximity of an old people's home. (Why do the traffic authorities persist with this stereotype?)

The pain increased, too, and in spite of visits to doctors (including an eminent one with consulting rooms near Harley Street), osteopaths, physiotherapists and other practitioners, it did not lessen. In fact it got worse. One day a friend of my mother's heard of my condition and brought me a book, Inside Yourself by Louise Morgan. It did not particularly impress me, but by that stage I was ready to try anything and this turned out to be a turning point in my life.

A few days later, I was entering a Victorian building in London, the consulting room of a dapperly dressed man of some fifty years. He was Patrick Macdonald, a teacher of the Alexander Technique. With very few preliminaries he asked me to sit down in a chair, not out of politeness but in order to study my manner of moving. In fact, I now suspect that he had already figured out the problem, and soon he was asking me to sit down again but this time to do it while following his instructions. He placed his hands on my neck as I moved and immediately stopped me. After a few attempts it seemed that I was totally unable to do as he wished. Instead of collapsing my body forwards and down into the chair as usual, he wanted me to direct my spine backwards and upwards as he took me to the chair. Again and again I failed before I was occasionally able to complete this task to his satisfaction.

Getting up was even worse – each time I tried to get out of the chair, the 'back and up' directions were countermanded by my well-entrenched habit patterns of 'forward and down'. Again and again I failed. This process continued daily for four weeks until I had to return to university.

Why did I continue to torture myself with failure in this way? There were two reasons. Firstly, something told me this man was right. I had been dimly aware that all was not well with the way I moved. A keen sportsperson, I had noticed that some aspects of my performance, for example at high jumping, were actually deteriorating at an age when they should have been improving. Maybe the AT teacher had the answer. Secondly, there was something about the way he himself moved that was more like the movement of a much younger man.

After more lessons in the summer vacation the pain started to lessen. I measured this by the fact that the time at which I just had to lie down became progressively later and later in the day. The morning was usually bearable but by lunch time verticality was usually a strain, particularly after sitting, something I had to do a lot of at university. I remember so well one evening when eventually I was able to stay up till midnight and another when I attended a sold-out performance of War and Peace and stood at the back of the cinema for four and a half hours! Finally, there came the day when I survived my first whole day spent on my beloved cricket field. It hurt a bit but it felt good.

It seems I had been in this state of combined tension and collapse as I played that squash game in 1959. No particular movement led to my pain. It was simply wear and tear. Certainly, X-rays showed two worn lumbar discs. But, as I came to learn, this did not come about by chance.

So what did I learn and how did the Alexander Technique influence my life?

Firstly, I learnt that it was possible to take charge of my life, initially just in terms of my body, but later in relation to more psychological aspects.

Secondly, as I applied the Technique to everyday acts, there was a progressive lessening of my pain. Initially I could only rescue myself from pain after it had started. But later it became possible to prevent it. I learnt to apply the Alexander Technique to walking, standing, sitting, eating, brushing teeth and so on. Yes, it was work, work on some of the most basic aspects of life. But the 'pay' was good, although I was not paid each week but only after some months and years.

Thirdly, there was a visible change in the way I moved. This visible change was not just something superficial which I was doing with my posture, but progressively there was an actual measurable change in my shape. Mostly, though, I felt in charge of an aspect of my life which had been in charge of me. My body changed into a more athletic shape and I began to stretch it into late nights, sport, postgraduate study, work, marriage, children and a 'normal' life.

Finally, this change in shape had the effect of making me more satisfied with the way I was and at ease with myself.

Now I believe that my relatively fit state at the age of sixty-six is due to practising this Technique. I have arranged a lifestyle which suits me, a basic working day from nine to four and a satisfying second career which has taken me all over the world.

Is this a fairy tale? A delusion? An illusion? Of course there are the difficulties of normal life. It is not all roses. But it is active and pretty fulfilled. So much for the personal. Is my account a fantasy? Is my improved condition objectively attributable to the Alexander Technique? In the final resort, who knows?

# Recognition of the Force of Habit

> *We get into the habit of performing a certain act in a certain way, and we experience a certain feeling in connexion with it which we recognise as 'right.' The act and the particular feeling associated with it become one in our recognition. If anything should cause us to change our conception, however, in regard to the manner of performing the act, and if we adopt a new method in accordance with this changed conception, we shall experience a new feeling in performing the act which we do not recognize as 'right.' We then realize that what we have hitherto recognized as 'right' is wrong.*
> *(Constructive Conscious Control, p. 131–2)*

The quotation above describes one of Alexander's main discoveries. What has become habitual seems normal to us, and what seems normal seems right. It is the nature of a habit that it can become locked in and resistant to change. This happens by means of a mechanism involving another of Alexander's concepts, that of unreliable sensory appreciation. (See "Unreliable Sensory Appreciation" on page 87.) The habits, mental and physical, which characterise the way we 'use' ourselves – the way we see and define ourselves – are fundamental. Our brain progressively becomes used to the chronic tensions associated with them. We are no longer in touch with our psychophysical state – what we really feel, what we really need, how we really are. Over time some habits may become counterproductive, even detrimental, and, worse still, resistant to change because of the sensations of normality embedded within them. The Alexander Technique offers a way of unlocking the force of habit and enabling change.

Dorothy Walker quotes from a diary written while having Alexander Technique lessons: 'I realise curling up into a ball to try to shut out the migraine pain was not a wise way to deal with it – for all those years! Even though, in my old age, I no longer have migraines the curling up habit is very hard to break.'

Theresa Turner, a musician trying to succeed in a competitive world, takes the habitual pain she encounters after practising long hours for granted, saying, 'I felt lost if I didn't have that habitual tension to work with'.

# The Fundamental Core of My Existence
## Clarissa Palmer

The Alexander Technique has changed my life in the most profound way imaginable. By luck I was introduced to an idea that has become the fundamental core of my existence. It imbues every moment of my life, for I have become physically mindful and am able to decide 'how to be'. I may not make the best choices, but at least I am aware that I am making them. Until I came upon the Technique I was a victim of my circumstances. At twenty-one, I had joined my father in the seemingly inevitable slipped-disc department (sharing the condition created a strange, yet pleasing, bond with him), as well as suffering from chronic indigestion and an excruciating hammer toe. Having suffered from undiagnosed glandular fever for two years, I was also weak and overtired. Since the age of thirteen, when I had grown six inches in six months, a droopy exhaustion was, for me, the norm.

Had I not had the great good fortune to have my first lesson in my early twenties I believe that I would still, thirty years later, be droopy and tired with that myriad of painful conditions that seem to beset so many of my middle-aged friends. I changed because I learned to think differently. I changed because, unenthusiastically at first, I understood that I needed to change. It took my poor teachers a great deal of patience and understanding to help me in my attempt to fulfil my potential. For this I am, and always will be, deeply grateful.

Never well coordinated as a young child, I became hopelessly incompetent when my growth spurt left me a dizzying six-foot tall in my early teens. Games was the worst part of every week, worse even than the endless teasing from fellow pupils and unpleasantness from a surprising number of teachers who felt inferior when addressing a taller pupil. I never stooped and was frequently praised for my excellent posture. What this meant was that I stood on one leg and dropped the other hip, creating many weird angles to compensate, collapsed internally but never, never rounded shoulders. The effect was, I was told, 'too romantic for words'; in reality it was an apologetic attempt to avoid physically dominating those around me. Modelling was suggested, half-heartedly, but I fell at the first casting couch hurdle by running away from an elderly agent who favoured nude romps in his office.

Eventually finding enjoyable employment in the theatre, I led a typical girl-about-town life, marred only by persistent lower-back pain, chronic indigestion and a painful toe that was awaiting surgery. I was blissfully unaware, at twenty-one, that there was an alternative approach.

Unable to stand for any length of time without pain, I went to a chemist and bought a corset – not a sexy basque, but a surgical garment full of metal reinforcement to hold up my sagging back – in the belief that this was the only way forward. I cycled every day, was slim and fit and had no idea why my back muscles could not support me. Wary of doctors since being treated for conditions I had never had, I refused pain relief and operations. Hence that hideous and uncomfortable corset: it was my version of self-help.

Luckily a random conversation over lunch with a friend changed my life. She had found the Alexander Technique. She bullied me into having a lesson, not because she remotely understood the benefits, but because she felt that I was bored and it would take my mind off my troubles. A work colleague, deeply concerned at the step I was taking, begged me to investigate further. He had heard that I would be obliged to lie with my head on some books, and that Alexander teachers believed that the texts would permeate my mind. At the very least, he insisted, I must check what books I was lying upon.

I arrived at my first lesson full of these bizarre concerns. Fate decreed that my teacher would be an Australian woman bursting with good humour, wisdom and down-to-earth common sense. The teacher had talents I little understood – what I would later realise were great 'hands' – and with them she coaxed and persuaded my body and (eventually) my mind to develop its own strengths. Crucially, she taught me to breathe.

I was a keen singer, taking lessons in opera, so I believed that breathing was my forte. It took a while for me to be persuaded otherwise. Now my greatest joy is to breathe and, as a tool to get through difficult times, it never fails. Events and ill health can temporarily knock the system about but, essentially, breathing freely is a lifesaver. It took me several years to realise this, as changing my physical habits felt 'wrong'. My friends saw the difference in me long before I could appreciate the transformation. The essential 'me' was being tampered with. I had to stop draping myself over any available surface and learn to stand on my own two feet.

My teacher admitted that my first visit had filled her with concern: I was like a long bit of overcooked spaghetti. Not a case for reducing undue tension, more a case of injecting a bit of life into this long, lax frame. Like a kind of Chinese water torture, she patiently repeated her instructions on a weekly basis. I often left full of embarrassment that she had had to repeat herself so often but, gradually, her message took root and I grew in strength and confidence.

The Alexander Technique filled me with wonder and admiration and, after a few years, I realised that I would love to train to be a teacher. I lacked the confidence to even suggest it. Thankfully, after many lessons, my teacher did. She felt that I had progressed well enough to consider training and believed that I had the qualities necessary to become a teacher. I had learnt to trust her judgement, so applied to become a student at one of the London schools. It is one of the best decisions I have made in my life.

At twenty-eight, nine months after having my first child, I started the three-year training course. It was pure joy despite the soul searching that change demands (I was too immature to enjoy it at first). The greatest hurdle, for me, was letting go of what I thought I already knew. I think I still find it the greatest challenge in all aspects of life. Coming from a position of physical weakness, I also found it trying to be tired again. It took me a long time to realise that tiredness does not always indicate weakness, but can be a sign of good work.

My strength had increased immeasurably since my first lessons. Now, my coordination improved too as I applied thought to activities previously too difficult to enjoy. I became a good skier once I realised that 'monkey' was the perfect position to be in, rather than the knock-kneed style I had previously favoured. A game of tennis was still tough, but at least I could hit the ball with the racket even if the direction and speed remained dodgy. My singing was transformed, partly by the Alexander Technique and partly by a change of singing teacher. I had always been asked to sing with 'a little more charm, dear', an instruction which crippled me with insecurity about my size and talent. Now I was told, 'That's an awful pissy sound for a woman of your size'. That idea, along with an application of good Alexander directions did the trick, and I have never stopped learning.

I took a part-time job as a textile conservator and was the only one in the workroom not to suffer from the tension and pain caused by the working conditions. Thinking about how I addressed the worktables – how I 'used' myself in the process – prevented any work-related injuries. Pregnancy and childbirth were wonderful opportunities to focus on 'use' and its benefits both to my babies and myself. The same is true of all activities: thoughtfulness prevents most problems from occurring. I found that with the help of the Technique I became aware of strain and stopped it before it created pain or damage. This is the tool (the ability to choose) that the Technique gave me.

One unforeseen consequence (at least by me) of the path I had chosen was that my height, keeping pace with my wellbeing, would increase. In F.M. Alexander's words, I was achieving my full height potential. I ran home and found that I had grown by an inch and a half. I was horrified, not stopping to think that this dead weight had been compressing my spine and stomach, thereby causing all my ills. Getting any taller was my worst nightmare. Had I been told at the start of the training course that the cost of a lifetime of understanding and improved health would be a fractional increase in height, I would have turned away and given up. The negative experiences I had suffered as a direct result of my height had been so unpleasant that I would not have been able to accept changing in that way.

Thankfully no one mentioned any such thing. I was allowed to grow both literally and emotionally so that, eventually, I was able to accept my height without too many concerns. Interestingly, my natural height, as opposed to the earlier collapsed version, elicited far less comment despite the extra inch. Good body language, another benefit.

The Alexander Technique is an ongoing process that continually enlivens every day. Responding to stimuli by thinking rather than reacting – whenever possible – is a process that keeps brain and body alert. Profound changes are possible with the smallest adjustments, often a form of controlled release that allows one's own potential to re-emerge.

I feel now that it is my Technique. With it I have been able to weather many storms. It has empowered me in a real sense, in that I have, if I wish, conscious control of what I am doing. It allows me to attempt to do my best – I haven't won Wimbledon, or sung at Covent Garden, but I have enjoyed improving my own performance. Insecure, collapsed, reactive, unmotivated, unable to sustain any activity for long – that was the young adult I had become. A chance encounter gave me the opportunity to change. It also gave me a legacy to pass on to my two children, born when the journey started. I will never cease to marvel at the luck that came my way and bless both my younger self for accepting the challenge and all my Alexander teachers, pupils and colleagues for facilitating the transformation.

## My Experience of the Alexander Technique as a Musician
Teresa Turner

I look around at my fellow musicians in the orchestra during a break in rehearsal. A cellist, slouched low in her chair, looking bored and uncomfortable. An oboist, also slumped – I wonder how he has any room to breathe at all. A violinist, jaw tightly clamped on the instrument, gaze fixed on the difficult passage of music he is practising, hardly taking a breath. I wonder, is this what music is about? As I stand there, I realise that not long ago I was in the same situation myself, and feel a certain sense of relief, almost smugness, that I have found a way out of the pain I thought I had to accept as part of being a musician, not to mention a double bass player, and not a tall one at that.

I started piano lessons at the age of twelve, followed by double bass at the age of fifteen. I was an eager learner, and joined my first orchestra after three months of bass lessons. It didn't take long for me to feel discomfort while playing, but I thought that that was something I had to put up with, not being tall (I'm five foot five inches). A double bass is taller than I am, with strings that are much thicker than guitar strings, that take a lot more finger strength to push down. I loved the bass from the start, so I decided to put up with it and keep playing anyway.

When I began playing in orchestras regularly, I would often do residential courses which involved playing up to nine hours a day. Needless to say, it didn't take long to feel the effects. For three years I had almost constant pins and needles across my left shoulder and back, as well as extreme tension in my hands and arms. Sometimes I would start to play and have to stop after five minutes because I would have so much pain in my arms, it felt like they were seizing up. To make a loud sound on the bass, for example, I thought that I had to really grip the bow and lean into the string. I had great difficulty in balancing the bass, not only when standing, but also while sitting, so the effort of stopping the instrument from falling, let alone playing, exacerbated that tension.

I had no patience for working at a piece for hours; instead I would attempt to play it up to speed straight away, not thinking about what the music was about but just reading the notes off the page. I wanted results straight away – I had no awareness of what I was doing with my body at the time, only of the black dots on the page in front of me. At the end of concerts, I would often be exhausted and hardly able to move my shoulders, and even sleep didn't help the discomfort go away; sometimes sleep made it worse. I never really told anyone about it, because I felt that people would just think I was making a fuss, or 'being a diva'. Being a female bass player, I felt like I had to prove myself, to show that I could do it too, that I was strong enough to stand up to the competition, that I wasn't 'just a girl'. As a result, I really pushed myself to try harder all the time to play better, and didn't give any thought to the effect it was having on my body.

When I finished school, I went on to do a four-year degree in music, with piano as my principal study. Practice rooms were hard to come by, so often I would wait until the evening and then play for up to two hours without a break. By the end of the practice session, I would be stiff and sore, especially in my shoulders and back. I very rarely warmed up before playing, not knowing then how important it was. Sometimes I would have so much pain in my hands and wrists I would tell my teacher, who recommended that I go for physiotherapy. I didn't like that idea, so I just ignored it and hoped the pain would go away by itself. Even though I knew that there were others like me who also suffered pain from overdoing it, I was still shy to mention it. I always felt that I had to put myself under pressure to improve my playing all the time, and found it extremely difficult not to compare myself to other people, considering that the piano is such a commonly played instrument and that there are so many brilliant players around. I had the belief that I had to 'do' something to make the music happen. 'Play musically!' and 'Relax your arms!' were instructions which I interpreted as 'Try harder!' and 'Make more effort!'

Finally, when I was nineteen, I was playing with an orchestra that had invited a teacher of the Alexander Technique to visit and teach us how to become more aware of ourselves when playing, how to use less effort and to relieve tension in performance. In my first meeting with her, she told me, 'I can see you've forgotten where your hip joints are!' My immediate reaction was to feel insulted – of course I knew where they were, it's my body! I quickly came to realise that, actually, I knew very little about how my body worked, apart from that I wasn't comfortable in it.

After that initial introduction, I started getting regular lessons with a teacher close to where I was studying and got such relief from it that I continued sessions on and off for about four years. I know that, especially early on in my experience of lessons, it was the physical release of tension, that 'relaxation', that made a significant impression on me. That release that I felt during hands-on work felt like such a relief – that one-to-one contact, so gentle and reassuring, giving me an opportunity to have time for myself. I felt lost if I didn't have that habitual tension to work with, almost as if there was no need for the lessons if it wasn't there. The more I learned however, the more I wanted to be able to share with others. It made so much sense, and brought together everything that I was interested in – how the body works, how people think, and how the two relate to each other. As a result, I made the decision to train to become an Alexander teacher myself, and am now in my final year.

I can safely say that without the Technique, I don't think I would still be playing today. As it is now, I have changed enormously in the last couple of years – I can now play the bass standing up, something I found impossible before due to my difficulty with balance (I always had to play while sitting on a high stool), and not only that but I can stay standing for an entire two-hour concert, no problem, with no pain. Instead of pushing into the string to make a big sound, I just allow the weight of my arm to draw the sound out. When I play piano, I find it so much easier now to learn new music. I find that I can be aware now if I do start to tense up at all and can stop before there is any pain. I am so much more in touch with what I am doing with my body while I play, instead of just focusing on the notes – and in turn, everything I play becomes more effortless, as if the music 'plays itself'.

My confidence in my ability as a musician has improved enormously. I find that the less I do, the easier everything has become. If I do feel

## Recognition of the Force of Habit

discomfort or pain, I no longer put up with it: I question why it's happening and change whatever it is that's causing it. Above all, I'm a much happier person, which in turn has made my music-making so much more rewarding and enjoyable. I have found the experience of learning the Alexander Technique to be hugely empowering – I've learned that I'm the one in charge of my own body, not the other way round!

# The Experience of an 'Older Person'
Dorothy Walker

My intention is to encourage people of my age (over seventy) not to be daunted by the habits of a lifetime. Uncovering and dealing with them can be fun and the results astonishing. I come from an era and a background where the body was a tool to get the work done. Taking up the idea of listening to my body and becoming at ease with it has given new energy to the later years of my life.

To give some little taste of the process, I went through a notebook which I have kept during my three years of lessons and what follows is a brief selection of my comments written there.

On rereading the little book, I am most forcibly struck by the immense patience of my teacher as I proudly (sometimes disconsolately) feed back my observations and discoveries, frequently rediscovering the same thing three months later! These habits and misuse, my teacher will have seen from the very beginning.

Here's your Christmas present – the money for your first Alexander lesson. But it was the beginning of March before I followed it up.

> *The first lesson's big question is, 'Why are you beginning Alexander lessons?'*

> *My answer, 'Because my friend urged me to', sounds weak, but it is true. Something to do with 'my shoulders being all hunched up with anxiety', I think the friend said.*

The other feature of the first lesson is being introduced to 'semi-supine', when of course I closed my eyes, as I do at other times in the lesson. In lesson two I learn that my eyes help balance by relating to verticals – don't close them.

My feet in contact with the ground also helps – it's recommended that I don't wear socks all the time. I'll just have to get used to the sight of my squashed, crunched up toes. Better still I could learn to wriggle them and they would improve and spread out.

The physical sensation of relaxation at the end of a lesson is great. However, by the end of the day my muscles complain bitterly about this 'releasing thing', i.e. they ache, a lot.

After about six lessons my confidence collapses: I can't do this, it is all too strange and unfamiliar. I am familiar with my thought processes and my brain; but my body? I don't like what I see in the mirror so it is very hard to work that way.

So we don't use the mirror.

Next lesson there is lots of encouragement given. Apparently it is quite usual to suffer lack of confidence, but it's a bit soon after only six lessons.

So I carry on.

My own thoughts later are that as I am in unfamiliar, even unknown territory, it is an adventure. Treat it that way! My reservations are that I am required to spend a lot of time thinking about myself, inhibiting, giving directions etc.(though these are not words I would have used then). But I probably spend a lot of time thinking about myself anyway. At least this is positive.

After a while I use a CD to guide me in my semi-supine. The first three bands are about twenty minutes each, so one band per semi-supine is helpful. Again the process and the terms used are a foreign language to me, but it keeps my eyes open(!) and gradually over the next few months of listening I get some understanding of the structure of my body.

> *I am creating a problem for myself, as I have this urge to finish the day's work before the semi-supine. Stopping in the middle is extremely difficult and yet I am one of the lucky people who could do so on most days. 'Preventative, not restorative' is a phrase to keep in mind. But it is so difficult to stop for 20 minutes even*

> *though the benefits are obvious when I do. If only I had known this seventy years ago!*

A new discovery is made. The right hand side of my body is much 'tighter' than the left. Now I can actually see this for myself, as I have learnt to focus in the mirror on a specific bit of myself. Thus I am not embarrassed, just interested.

Having read some sections of *Job's Body*, I am amazed at the intricacy of connection between muscles and nerve cells etc. No wonder I feel different. The lesson sessions are not about emotions, but muscle release is. Once it has been pointed out it is obvious that the release of tension built up over so many years is going to be felt not just physically but emotionally as well. Sometimes when I get home after a lesson I only want to sit in the garden and not even think.

I realise curling up into a ball to try to shut out the migraine pain was not a wise way to deal with it – for all those years! Even though, in my old age, I no longer have migraines the curling up habit is very hard to break.

> *Another 'curling' habit I have discovered is wrapping my feet round the chair legs. I seem never to sit with my feet squarely on the floor – but then I don't stand squarely either.*

> *Am I standing comfortably? If I am, then I need to correct my right foot, which will be turned outwards, twisting the right knee which is the one that hurts when I go upstairs.*

> *The Alexander Technique isn't just a thing one does sometimes, it is a way of life. Half measures won't do and you can't cheat (yourself).*

We have a review at the end of two years, and what I find I have gained is confidence. For someone in their seventies that is surely quite an achievement. Also, physically I am more supple, and I enjoy the feeling. (More supple than some of my contemporaries who have always been athletic.)

After a few more months it dawns on me that I don't want to hold my head up when walking or meeting people. It is so contrary to my lifelong philosophy of 'keep your head down and get on with it'. Decision time! Do I now cease being an Alexander pupil?

What has happened to my newly found confidence?

Over the next few weeks I come to acknowledge that it is my frightened thoughts and emotions that have the 'head down' philosophy. My body quite likes being 'open' and I think wisdom lies there, rather than in my usual negative attitude.

Confidence restored.

It feels like I am at the beginning all over again, but not quite, because I now know the sensation of being 'all of a piece' sometimes after a lesson or even, for a fleeting moment, on other occasions. That sensation is worth the struggle, which I shall enjoy continuing.

## Council Worker, Speech Therapist
Sean Richardson

I am a forty-year-old city council worker and newly qualified speech and language therapist. About ten years ago, I had this vague nascence of awareness of the fact that I experienced stress, and that it was reflected in my body. I was aware that I was probably more stressed than I needed to be for the circumstances I was in. I read something about the Alexander Technique in a magazine or somewhere, which explained that it was looking at the conjunction of mind and body (if, indeed, you can make that separation to start with). I was aware of over-breathing – a tendency to breathe shallowly. I came more from a general understanding of the fact that there was some sort of link between psychological and physical states, and I wanted to learn how to control those a little better.

Earlier, I had had some pain at the top of my back and my GP had advised the Alexander Technique, but I hadn't got the money to pay for it at the time. I also sprained my back doing press-ups. I was doing a delivery job and was in and out of the car twenty-five times a day, and would sometimes strain my back.

I struggled with the idea of 'non-doing'. Using the Alexander Technique always does me noticeable good, whenever I practise the lying down. I'm constantly scanning at the same time as attending to whatever I'm listening to, e.g. music. I always notice when I get up a lightness in my body and a sort of fluidity in my movements. I'm 'resetting' on a regular basis, at least five times a week.

I can't really say that I regularly use it carrying out all activities. My attention is drawn too much by the task. I'm able to notice occasionally, when I'm in a social situation specifically, that I'm tightening my jaw and the shallow breathing starts. In fact, it's not just the jaw, the whole of my body tightens up, and I would be really trying to force my conversation out when I'm with pretty much anyone I don't know very well. I try and control that but I still have a lot of difficulty. It still feels to me like becoming aware and giving the directions takes up too much of my brain's processing power!

When it comes to doing sort of general physical activities, I'm afraid I don't really use it that much, but I'm wondering whether to a certain extent, I probably adapted to the level of ability that I've got. So it always feels like I could be doing more, but, during that last ten years, I've probably progressed quite a long way anyway so I don't want to make it sound like I don't use it at all because I think I probably do.

I thought about coming back for a few more lessons, perhaps about five years ago, but I made a rash decision to go back to university; so really I've had to draw in my horns financially.

I have very little back pain or neck problems these days. I still have a little bit of a back problem at the very bottom right hand side from something that happened during the time that I had lessons. I went over to India; I did a meditation course and damaged my sciatic nerve. I went to an osteopath and three years ago went to a McTimoney chiropractor. I can't say either really noticeably helped, but strangely, things have gradually got better. It was never severe pain, it was discomfort, more a sort of pins and needles, electric shock-type thing down the back of the leg. Sitting cross-legged for more than about a minute was out, because that would cause problems. About three years ago I went to a wedding at a Sikh Gurdwara where you have to sit cross-legged for quite a long time. What I noticed was that by sitting there for awhile cross-legged, then standing up, and then moving it around, things sort of opened up on their own; so I went back to sitting cross-legged occasionally and working it up. Now I'm in the position where I'm not getting too much bother from it at all.

Over the course of the last few years several people have remarked positively on my posture. I had the reputation for being the most upright-seated person in the office. Everyone used to joke about how I wasn't doing any work but at least I looked good. One bloke that I worked with recently was always going on about it, and I remember seeing him in town and he said 'I knew it was you from a distance, I recognised the posture'.

I used to be something of a sloucher. I met an ex-girlfriend. I was eighteen when I was going out with her. I was about three stone lighter with long hair, but she said I seemed taller, and I wasn't slumped over. That might be partly to do with becoming more self-confident anyway, but I'm convinced that the Technique has had more than fifty percent input into that. I just wasn't aware, as most people aren't, of what I was doing with myself. And it has made me a lot more aware of my psychophysical state. I think I was someone who was always given to being quite introspective, but it has helped make my awareness more acute.

I do use it, not as much as I would like, but I do use it, in social settings. I go to the gym and I think it is essential that I don't hurt myself working out. I don't do anything that I know is going to put strain on in the wrong way, so all in all, I think it has had some major benefits, physical and emotional.

I can't think of anything bad about the Alexander Technique. It might be said that it's made me more neurotic, less spontaneous in a sense, but I don't personally agree, because I reckon what other people call 'spontaneity' is just their automatic habitual reaction and not very spontaneous at all.

When I used to run, I would get knee pains. I now run an average of four times a week, and I get no aches and pains because I do use the Technique.

It is certainly fair to say that tendrils of Alexander Technique unfolded to all parts in my life, like with the running. It's made me very aware that even when I'm completely on my own, there's still these constantly flowing currents of attention, to see how they are linked with what I'm thinking about at the time.

My dissertation for my speech therapy course was about stuttering, and I have noticed that after running, my own fluency would actually be improved for a while, from running while using the Alexander Technique, so I was sort-of interested in the psychophysical aspects and I did read some papers that related to the Alexander Technique and stuttering. I think you can say that physically it's benefited me, psychologically it's benefited me and intellectually as well, as I've used some of the insights that I have gained to apply to the dissertation that I wrote, and to talk about the mind/body continuum.

# Why I Study the Alexander Technique
## Dorothy Jerrome

I came to the Alexander Technique six years ago in search of an effective therapy for my husband, who suffered from Parkinson's disease. We had read a research report in which the AT had had the most beneficial outcomes for this illness, in comparison with other therapies. Our hopes were justified, and for a year my husband visibly unfolded in his weekly sessions, though the effects did not last much beyond the lessons. He adored the teacher and clearly benefited from the one-to-one, hands-on approach. The effort of attending weekly lessons, despite the short-term gains, proved too much and we stopped them after about a year.

After a few months, I found I was missing my own lessons and decided to return. Four years on, I am more involved than ever. I have come to value the AT for all sorts of reasons – physical, emotional, aesthetic, philosophical and intellectual.

As I understand it, the central message of the AT is that action ideally involves releasing, undoing, letting go, using minimum effort to accomplish physical tasks. I have found this to be emotionally gratifying and physically very helpful, unlike the sweat and strain of other body work like yoga, or even the stretching and bracing involved in dance.

The AT approach to movement reminds me constantly to be in the moment, avoiding the tendency to arrive – a lifetime habit. I like the conceptual neatness of it, the idea of three options: to carry on as before, to do nothing, or to do something different. I find my teacher's images helpful – to go along the familiar path, not to go at all, or to create a new path so that this becomes the familiar one and the old path is overgrown and disappears.

The Technique is also intellectually challenging. There is a paradoxical struggle to hold onto the perspective of freedom from effort, while releasing: thinking … but not too much! There is always something to work at, something more to learn, some aspect of movement I have not thought of before, or which has emerged as an issue in the course of the previous week. When I was caring for my husband the problems I brought to my lessons concerned lifting and pushing, endlessly picking things up, cleaning and accessing high shelves, dealing with the physical and emotional strains of caring. I am still concerned with problematic tasks: driving with painful hands, carrying heavy objects, sitting down uncomfortably in my Quaker meeting and so on. I've appreciated my teacher's flexible and creative response to the issues I bring and have come to regard her as a friend and confidante as well as a guide to the workings of my body.

I find the philosophy of AT very congenial. The notion of the core of our being as stillness, the need for a pause between thought and action, the importance of space – between my movements, between my joints, between my thoughts – are ideas which find a strong resonance with my Quaker beliefs and sacred dance which I practise passionately. Sacred dance involves the idea of a mandala in motion, discovery of the still point of the turning world, the notion of opening the heart. I have found in the AT a powerful reinforcement of the idea of trusting the process of opening up.

There is also a correspondence between these ideas with a third area of passionate involvement – with the natural world, which I approach partly through botanical drawing and painting. The quietness and openness encouraged by the AT makes me think of the combination of stillness and intense movement in nature, and of ourselves as part of the natural world.

My art is one aspect of a very visual approach to life. Not surprisingly, I derive aesthetic satisfaction from the AT. I love the beautiful stance of the natural body. I value the child-like form we have in mind when we think of the directions, a form unspoiled by fashion or the requirements of modern, adult living.

I recently experienced the joy of a more intense AT experience at a school in a couple of three-hour sessions shared with students of the Technique. I see that training at this level can create a sense of physical meditation: calming, uplifting and rejuvenating. I am sad that I discovered that too late, but I hope to continue my AT journey in another setting.

A major feature of the AT experience for me has been that of learning from a teacher. As a hands-on practice, there has been a meeting of bodies and minds. More than that, my long association with my teacher through the weekly lessons has become a very comfortable experience, a sharing of thoughts and perspectives on life which has sustained me through difficult times. My teacher's example of physical comfort, *joie de vivre* and a wonderful lightness of being makes her a great advertisement for the Alexander Technique!

# Reflections
## Janette Griffin

I was born in 1955, the year that F.M. Alexander died. This may be an insignificant coincidence, but I believe that destiny has urged me to follow his footsteps for reasons that are constantly unfolding. Now in my fifty-sixth year, I feel a desire to explore what has led me to follow this journey and how it has helped me. A circuitous route through life's rich tapestry has often felt like a maze with no exit. Studying the work of Alexander has encouraged me to accept the randomness of life. More importantly, it has enabled me to recognise that I now have a choice of how to react to its unpredictability.

Recommended reading on Alexander training courses are books by the man himself, including his second work *Constructive Conscious Control of the Individual*. This contains a slightly uninviting section entitled 'Psycho-Physical Equilibrium'. Trying to unravel Alexander's writing style can sometimes be challenging, but like Shakespeare it can ultimately be very rewarding. Within this section, I was to find the clearest understanding of my journey to date.

At the age of twenty-three, I spent three weeks in hospital following complete loss of coordination (unable to carry out any normal activities: walking, eating and so on). Various tests (including a very unpleasant lumbar puncture) confirmed a diagnosis of multiple sclerosis. This was all very frightening, and viewed as 'something terrible that was happening to me'. It became all too easy to consider myself a victim of outside circumstances.

In actual fact, my sense of victimhood had probably begun much earlier, following childhood events outside my control. Psychologically, this left me expecting the worst to happen. Worse, I came to almost expect that this would continue. After reading Alexander's section on psycho-physical equilibrium, the most significant contribution toward this I now believe to be as follows.

Memories of an earlier period in hospital at the age of nine had been successfully suppressed and seemed very insignificant. My right knee had given way during a school game of rounders, and involved an operation for suspected cartilage trouble (pre-keyhole surgery; I am left with a scar of six inches, often mistaken for laddered stockings!). As in Alexander's example, I had to re-learn how to walk 'properly' (overseen by mannequin mother and Air Force father, both with their own ideals). I have memories of mother trying her best to soak off Elastoplast from thigh to calf. It was similar to slow, painful exfoliation. Meanwhile, father was left to supervise seemingly endless walks back and forth on the upstairs landing, encouraging me not to 'limp'.

My 'successful' learning how to walk again involved many emotional factors, most notably wanting to get it 'right', fear of looking 'odd' and a desire to please parents. At the time they were going through marital problems, resulting in divorce a few years later. I will be ever grateful to them, for they did the best they could in the circumstances.

How I wish, though, that the Alexander Technique had been available to me at this time. I firmly believe the operation and life events (and my own reaction to these) to be the cause of my dis-ease. I am not denying the diagnosis of MS, or looking for 'something out there' to explain it. I am suggesting that there is more to life than a 'diagnosis', whatever it may be. The worst does not have to happen and if it does, so be it. Nothing in life is guaranteed, much as we humans try to make it so. Ultimately, the Alexander Technique has taught me that my victimhood is no longer required, replacing it with curiosity and wonder at all of life's peaks and troughs.

Since the initial onset of MS symptoms in 1978, my dis-ease had followed a relapsing/remitting course with intermittent disabling attacks. Various medical interventions have included steroids, removal of all amalgam fillings, calcium tablets, muscle relaxants, anti-depressant medication (stopped in 2005) and, from 2001, alternate daily injections of the disease-modifying drug Betaferon (which I chose to stop in December, 2010).

My interest in the Alexander Technique began around 2005, when it was suggested by my reflexologist. Having lessons and reading around the subject inspired me to pursue this avenue further.

It is certainly difficult to define exactly what the Alexander Technique is, but could our constant search for definitions (or recognisable 'boxes') be part of the problem? The Alexander Technique is not a patient/therapist relationship but more a re-education process between student/teacher, with a specific syllabus of 'unlearning' bad habits. It is possible that such habits, perhaps originally acquired to avoid physical and/or psychological discomfort, are no longer proving useful and could even be detrimental to our overall wellbeing.

I feel that the Alexander Technique allows individuals to regain a belief that they have some control (however small) over their situation through awareness, and that they are free to choose their response. Rather than just accepting problems as something that happen 'to' us and seeing ourselves as victims, the Alexander Technique encourages us to explore further and adopt a proactive approach to help ourselves as much as possible. This sense of 'doing' (even if only by altering negative thought patterns) can in itself provide motivation and a sense of achievement.

> My own improvements include:
> Freedom from headaches
> Improved sleeping
> More stamina
> Noticeably improved balance
> Better walking (and running!)
> Improved sensory awareness
> Less stress
> More confidence
> Breaking habits of negative thinking
> Freedom from drug dependency
> Freedom from fear

The Alexander Technique has enabled me to take responsibility for my own wellbeing, preventing me from returning to 'victimhood' and seeking something or someone out there to blame. I began attending a training course in 2007 on a part-time basis while still working. Three years later I was able to become a full-time student of the Alexander Technique, following the death of both parents and a modest inheritance. Perhaps it is the best tribute I can give them.

# The Long Road to the Carriage-Driving Trials Championship
Karen Scott-Barrett

As a child, I did a great deal of horse riding and was competing a lot by the age of nineteen, but I suffered from extreme and constant hip and back pain, and was therefore advised to give up riding at that time, which I did; however the pain did not disappear.

When I was twenty-nine, after many years of physical problems and even difficultly with walking and sleeping because of pain, I was finally diagnosed with multiple epiphyseal displasia and osteochondritis dissecans which, in simple terms, means hereditary malformation of the joints and damage to joints due to lack of blood supply. I was told by various consultants and doctors at the time that nothing could really help these conditions, that I must be careful never to put on too much weight and never to do any strenuous exercise. They said that I would certainly suffer from early-onset osteoarthritis and that I would need hip replacements before I was forty.

In my early thirties, I was suffering from such severe and debilitating bouts of neck pain, in addition to the continuing hip and lower-back pain, that I again visited a consultant, who told me that I had two severely prolapsed discs in my neck and that I was on the verge of paralysis – in fact he said that just tripping while walking could leave me permanently paralysed. He said that immediate surgery was essential, although he warned me that there was a fifty percent possibility that I might be left paralysed by the operation. I had two very young children and was extremely worried about who would look after them during the time I would be in hospital, and also during the long months of rehabilitation necessary if the operation was successful. So I delayed the operation while I thought about this.

Meanwhile an osteopath had suggested that I look into the Alexander Technique, although when he heard my consultant's diagnosis he urged me to take his advice and have an immediate operation. Nevertheless,

I found a teacher and started weekly lessons immediately, despite thinking it couldn't possibly be of much help, given the severity of my problems.

Much to my amazement, I started to feel better and the neck pain began to disappear. The pain in my lower back and hips also began to ease somewhat. To my consultant's extreme disapproval, I continued to put off the operation on my neck despite him telling me it was not possible for me to recover from severely prolapsed discs without surgery. After a year, he finally agreed that I need not come back to visit him until my next attack of neck pain, which he assured me was bound to occur because I could not really have recovered. I have never been back to see him, nor have I had any operations since except to pin a broken arm.

After a year of regular lessons, I went on to train as an Alexander teacher and I experienced enormous relief from my almost lifelong pain as a result of learning the Alexander Technique. I had not realised that I held extreme tension throughout my body all the time, and learning how to let go of this tension and how to use my body in a better way produced a remarkable improvement in my physical and also my mental state. It truly was life transforming and I am enormously grateful for everything the Alexander Technique has taught me: I have become infinitely more relaxed and positive as a person and able to cope much more easily with any problems and challenges I encounter.

Aged forty-nine, I had some X-rays done of my spine and major joints. I was told I had no signs of any prolapsed discs in my neck, nor of arthritis in any of my joints, although there was obvious malformation and signs of wear and tear in my hip joints. I have a very active life now and suffer from remarkably little pain. I still can't really ride, but I do have horses again, and for the last five years I have hugely enjoyed competing in carriage-driving trials, which involves lots of course-walking and general physical activity.

I passed my Class 1 Large Goods Vehicle driving test and now I drive an eighteen-tonne truck and trailer. I find my Alexander training enormously useful for my driving technique and posture (both truck and carriage driving) and for any nervousness I might have about competing, and I feel it contributes much to my success – I have even been National Champion in horse-driving trials. I think extraordinary things are possible with belief, and the help of the Alexander Technique!

# Using the Alexander Technique in Liturgy and Teaching
## Father Alcuin Schachenmayr

The Alexander Technique has helped me to grow as a monk, teacher and priest. My responsibilities as a Cistercian monk can vary greatly in the course of a single day, but I find my weekly Alexander lesson helps me in the liturgy, in public speaking and the many hours I spend at my desk every day with study, prayer and computer work. I've been studying in Vienna for the past six years; the work my teacher and I do together is very flexible. I bring along concerns from my daily life and sometime even the objects or texts with which I work.

Feelings of exhaustion after teaching a long class or presiding at two Sunday Masses prompted me to take up contact with an Alexander teacher. I had had a good experience as a student of the Technique while at university. Resuming lessons after a ten-year break, I soon found that my liturgical activity and public speaking became more creative. With the Technique, not only the musical and rhetorical aspects, but also the use of myself were now opened up to creative choices. I discovered a new domain of control where before I had been struggling along with habitual tension and strain. I experienced more choices during preaching and liturgical movement, making these assignments even more rewarding to me.

As a teacher, I sometimes lecture up to four hours a day. That's a challenge to physical endurance, when you consider that I have about four hours of liturgical prayer a day. Through the Alexander Technique I started to gain more control over my voice, and that made me feel more relaxed and playful while speaking in public. Since I find it crucial to stand and move while lecturing, I used to get tired fast. The Technique has changed that and made me lighter. That helps attract concentration from my listeners!

Monks in the Christian tradition live in a close connection between study and prayer; in reading sacred texts (lectio divina), what begins as study soon goes over into the realm of meditation. This means that even the way we sit at a desk can have a major effect on our thinking – and our prayer. Bad use of our selves leads to less creative thinking and, yes, less openness to the working of the Holy Spirit.

Most monks living in the twenty-first century need to communicate with others using the same media that everyone else uses: cell phones, emails, computer databases, Facebook. Since a monk has given his whole life to God and the Church, even his administrative work will have a religious dimension. He counsels the faithful, but even quotidian contacts with others should be pastoral; we believe every person is an image of God, every single person is worth the price Christ paid for him or her on the Cross. So the choices, creativity and sense of recollection I gain though the Alexander Technique make a difference in everyday contacts, too: they help to set the appropriate tone, even in difficult situations where patience wears thin. Good use makes for improved communication skills.

The most beautiful work a priest has to do is administering the sacraments. Here, God works through the priest to grant grace and comfort to believing Christians. Of course, the Alexander Technique changes nothing whatsoever about that theological fact, yet if the people involved practise good use of themselves, they will experience these moments in a more profound way. Two examples should clarify my point: a priest hearing confessions in a cramped, hunched-over way will distract from the beauty of this sacrament. Secondly, a priest baptising an infant while clutching various vessels (and the infant!) while he works, will experience the spiritual rebirth of the baby in a merely theoretical way.

My last point concerns liturgical space. Cistercian architecture is famous for its dramatic perspectives, in which severe simplicity is made vibrant through a dramaturgy of light. I belong to Heiligenkreuz Monastery near Vienna, an abbey famous for Romanesque architecture and soaring Gothic spires. To remain aware of the remarkable spaces in which I am privileged to pray and work requires inner discipline. So I apply principles of the Alexander Technique to practise widening my peripheral vision: I let my weight go down through the floor and back and up into the high-arched ceiling to experience the vertical dimension. Liturgical life is full of movement; the Technique also helps with processions, moving through crowded churches, even dealing with occasional disruptions that are part of liturgical life.

My experience shows that the Alexander Technique is remarkably well-suited to a monk's daily life; to be honest, I hadn't thought it would pervade so many aspects of my day. Surprising discoveries keep coming, and that makes me grateful I decided to stick with it all these years.

# Inhibition

> *This is an indirect procedure, and, as has already been shown, it involves the inhibition of familiar messages responsible for habitual familiar activity, and the substituting for these of unfamiliar messages responsible for new and unfamiliar activity.*
> *(The Universal Constant in Living, p. 12)*

> *But instead of employing inhibition, he adds to his difficulties by renewing his efforts on the old basis to put right what he is told is wrong, and he actually employs increased force in accordance with his own estimate of the amount needed to perform the act. And why so? Chiefly because the ordinary human being has lost the habit of inhibition, and because he is guided here by his sense of feeling, in this connection the most unreliable guide. (Man's Supreme Inheritance, p. 158)*

The Alexandrian sense of the word *inhibition* should be distinguished from the rather negative one which has become lodged in popular usage. It refers, simply, to a restraint on habitual, unthinking reaction. The process is a two-stage one. Firstly, we need to make a pause in our activities; we then need to identify and prevent any harmful habit associated with the action we are about to undertake.

Keith Hawkins, who describes himself as 'a rather excitable sort of chap' with difficulty speaking, says that if he forgets to pay attention his voice 'goes pear-shaped'. 'I must,' he says, 'remind myself to momentarily STOP talking, allow my breathing to normalise, relax my palate and use Alexander directions to regain my composure.'

Far from being restrictive, it becomes a liberating influence. Helen May, occasionally ambushed by 'emotional gusts' in her Alexander Technique teacher training as she releases physical tension, learns to recognise these gusts as 'yet another stimulus, yet another opportunity to inhibit and direct'. In our stories, saying 'no' to habitual patterns of response opens up a range of unexpected possibilities.

# The Twelve Pound Tale
## Helen May

Twelve pounds? Really? As in 12lb!

That's almost a stone, I think, as I am handed the heavy cake tin full of metal kitchen weights. That is the approximate weight of a human head, this lady tells me. Turns out she is a teacher of something called the Alexander Technique, and so I begin without even knowing it.

Looking back after twelve years, one for every pound in that tin, it is easier to chart my journey, but at the time it just sort of unfolded. I am a teacher of the Technique now, and this is my story.

So there I am, in 1998, standing in a school hall at a local practitioners' event, hearing about this Alexander Technique. I am an active mum with a young daughter, part-time job, and home and garden to run. So busy, busy, busy. As I hold this really heavy tin, I am struck by the idea that maybe carrying and balancing this heavy head of mine might have something to do with my continuous back and neck pain? Hum, sounds plausible to me.

I am used to pain: old injuries from training as a classical ballet dancer with shin splints and bloody toes from pointe work, considered normal and dismissed. Years of working as a stage manager in theatres, pushing heavy scenery around and working very long hours. I've loved it all, but the cost has been visiting chiropractors to ease the pain in my back when it gets too bad. That works for a while, until the next time I can hardly move.

Then there are new injuries from rushing around, carrying kids, bikes and groceries. My gardening and vegetable growing become increasingly difficult as the pain in my back and neck intensifies, as do my visits to the chiropractor.

I consult the medics, and eventually MRI and X-rays reveal that I have structurally damaged my sacroiliac joints and some of the vertebrae in my neck. Uh-oh, I think, I'm only thirty-eight years old for goodness' sake and yet I can't do a lot of things I want to, simply because I hurt too much. I am offered pain killers and anti-inflammatory drugs. This really worries me: what will I be like in ten, twenty or thirty years' time? There is talk of surgery in the future to fuse vertebrae to reduce the wear and tear on my spinal nerves. I really do not want to sentence myself to a life of pain and restricted movement, but what else is there?

I realise I have vaguely heard of the Alexander Technique, in passing, as I work in theatres. I thought it was for actors only, not me, as it was something to do with improving voice projection or posture, wasn't it?

Apparently not, as it turns out, or perhaps I should say that those outcomes may be by-products of the Technique over time but they are not the core – more of that later.

Suffice it to say, I am sufficiently intrigued by what I am hearing about the Alexander Technique to take up this teacher's offer of an introductory course she is going to run locally for a small group of us mums. Great, I think, I can squeeze that into my schedule too.

We have a good time. It's fun to learn about something new, and to begin to see and accept that the way I am using my body, every day, is linked to how well or not I am able to function and do things. So I am excited, as the Technique seems to be offering me a way to help myself – and it does. I have lessons on and off for the next five years. They help with pain reduction and a freer range of movement and I love it. However I feel as if I am missing something important, and slowly I understand that I am using the Technique to enable myself to do more and more and more. Great, you might think, but really, I am just pushing myself harder and harder. I haven't understood that what I really need to do first is to stop.

I know that I want to train to be a teacher of the Technique but how can I fit it in and afford it? I have my part-time job, teaching stage management to drama students during the week. I am in the middle of my PGCE in post-compulsory education. So, I start by doing an Alexander training course that is run over a weekend once a month. Sure, I can fit that in. I manage most of the first year, and it is interesting and valuable stuff, but I realise that I need a different approach. I allow myself to be easily distracted by my busy life and I am not disciplined enough to practise by myself. I need the structure, time and self-permission that training every day will give me.

It dawns on me that I need this to be my life, not something I squeeze into it. This is a personal choice to change my part-time training to a full-time course. It takes time for me to finish my PGCE and negotiate with my family and employer to make this possible. I really enjoy my job and need it to help pay for my training. My teaching timetable is changed, freeing up my mornings, and I am now able to start a three-year course in September 2005. Hurrah!

So, here I am on my first morning, standing in another hall with a group of fellow students and our head of training. I'm keen as mustard and ready to learn. It is very quiet in this lovely, spacious room. In fact, it is unnervingly quiet. I glance around and everyone seems very composed, but when will we start?

Now, I am the first to admit that I am a great 'doer' and a pragmatist through and through. I always want to know what something is for or how something is going to work. How it is going to make a difference to something or someone, preferably for the better? And, you know what, I want to know now, so can we please get on with it? My poor teacher, he is infinitely patient with me as I fight to be a 'good' student for a very long time.

I slowly discover that this learning is so different from what I thought learning was. I actually have to do less, very bizarre for someone with a strong work ethic. I find myself thinking, what do you mean when you say 'less is more'? That just doesn't make sense, perhaps if I try harder? Nope, that really doesn't work, as I get tenser and tenser. But I want to get it right, to be a good student: that's the way I was raised.

To start with I am easily frustrated with myself, with the Technique, with my teachers and with the writings of F.M. Alexander. It all seems so dense, so opaque, so wordy and takes a lot of digesting. Over the three years I eventually relish becoming a detective about myself and F.M.'s books. Reading, discussing, arguing with colleagues and going back to his book *The Use of the Self*, and myself – again and again.

I begin to understand that I need to give up my preconceived ideas not only about myself but about how I function. It turns out that my internal body-map is anatomically incorrect. I am not made the way I thought I was. Where does this heavy head of mine actually attach to my neck? Knowing structurally how I am constructed, where my joints really are and how they are designed to work helps me to function better. I enjoy the changes that our studies in anatomy bring to my thinking and moving.

I often find myself laughing as I come up against myself and all my powerfully ingrained habits. What do you mean you expect me to be able to walk from here? Are you kidding? I can't do that, as I am not starting from my familiar place nor getting ready in my usual or habitual way. I walk anyway and learn that it is possible after all. So there is not a correct position for me to be in, but only a correct condition of being consciously present. I love being in class, finding myself sitting down or standing or walking with no familiar idea of how I got there. How exhilarating that so little effort was involved, how scary that I don't feel like me anymore – help! I am beginning to learn to stop interfering with my system. When I am able to do this, my system can function the way it is designed to without all the extra interference I unconsciously like to add in.

This work seems full of paradoxes, and I find I am often surprised by how inaccurate my feelings are. I can feel like I am leaning forwards when a quick glance in the mirror shows me the opposite. How strange, talk about faulty sensory perception, so often the opposite of what I feel is what is actually happening. My desire to feel things out, and then make a judgement call as to how well I am doing, is a difficult thing to give up. After all, my senses are constantly giving me feedback and it is hard to simply notice without reacting. I want to follow my thoughts, my directions into my body, but in doing so I realise I am interfering with myself rather that getting out of my own way.

## Inhibition

Talking of feelings, I am occasionally ambushed by my release of emotional tension as I let go of a physical one, and find myself crying. Somehow they got stored together in my musculature and movement. I am beginning to understand why F.M. called them 'emotional gusts', and gusty they can be. I learn not to panic or feel embarrassed. They will pass. I recognise that here is yet another stimulus, yet another opportunity to inhibit and direct. Or not. In the end, it is always my choice.

Finally, I understand that it all comes down to my freedom to choose how I react to what comes at me, either from the outside or the inside. I find that inhibition is a real gift, especially to a workaholic like me. As far as I know, it is distinctive to the Technique, and for me inhibition is at the core. I think it is tricky to describe inhibition in words, as it is an experience unique to each individual, and each of us will make our own meaning. I will have a go anyway. I would say inhibition is when I consciously make a space between a stimulus and my response. It is very creative, because in that space, between noticing and doing, I am able to make an informed choice instead of reacting automatically. I get off the treadmill of my unconscious habits for a while.

Staying with the subject of definitions, I find I am often asked, 'What is the Alexander Technique?' I have come to appreciate that it is quite hard to answer this question, because the Technique is so experiential. However, for what it is worth, I think the Alexander Technique is the study and conscious experience of thinking in relation to movement.

Now I am fifty years old and rarely experience pain, despite my active life and burgeoning vegetable garden. I am a teacher of the Technique; I still go into class once a week and I also have a new part-time job which I've organised around my Alexander life, rather than the other way round.

Was it easy? Yes and no. There were considerable costs involved. Costs in terms of money, certainly more than twelve pounds. Costs in terms of time and balancing my commitments to family, work and life in general. Then there were costs to myself in learning to accept, and eventually delight in, the unknown, the uncomfortable and the sometimes downright terrifying experience of change. Luckily I had great companions along the way: encouraging teachers, other supportive students and eventually pupils. It is a privilege to be and work alongside them all.

In the end, I want to say thank you to Frederick Matthias Alexander for his Technique and especially the gifts of inhibition and direction. I have learnt to endgain less, to be more reflective and not such a 'doer'. Oh, I have aspirations and goals, it's just that now I care about how I reach them, rather than rushing blindly without paying attention to the process. I realise this work is not a quick fix, but it can be a lasting one if I am willing to do what Alexander did and begin again every day, starting afresh with those basic principles of stopping, thinking and choosing. And so this has become a life sentence after all, one that I welcome, one that I enjoy.

# My Journey to the Alexander Technique, Surgery and Beyond
Mary Rawson

I was about eight or nine years old when I first began to realise that what I was experiencing was back pain. I didn't know there was a problem except that I had difficulty keeping up with the family when out walking. My legs hurt but I didn't know any different; to me it was normal. I was a bit of a tomboy, having three brothers, and I enjoyed all the sports on offer at school. When rolling on my back on a hard gym floor I felt a 'knobble' low in my back that got in the way.

At around age thirteen my parents became worried. I kept holding onto my back and rubbing it, and I started to complain about pain. The doctor said I would probably grow out of it and that it was probably to do with a growth spurt. The orthopaedic surgeon said he could operate but that I may not be any better off. So there was no decision to be made. The general medical opinion was that I would have to learn to live with it. This was the motto I grew up with. I had a corset made to minimise the movement in my low back, but it made the whole situation worse. Eventually, with a lot of teenage disgust, the corset was binned.

I had a condition called spondylolisthesis (literally meaning slippage of a vertebra) due to the fracture or malformation of the bits of bone that support the little joints between the lumbar vertebrae, leaving the lower lumber vertebra slipped forward on the sacrum. Because of this fracture, the posterior process (the 'knobble') of the vertebra jutted out at the back. The cause of this condition can either be congenital or due to accident: in my case it was congenital. The potential of the disc between the vertebrae being impinged causing irritation to the sciatic nerve was high, causing leg pain and inevitably low-back pain. I was advised to stop sport and gymnastic activities, which I loved, including my favourite hobby, horse riding. I was not entirely obedient to this rule but it did curtail what I was used to doing. I now carried the label 'bad back', and I must admit it did become a bit of an excuse at times for not doing things that I could or should have done. I was having difficulty 'learning to live with it'.

'If only I could find someone who could fix my back then I could get on with the rest of my life', was my overriding thought. In my late teens and twenties all sorts of other discomforts arose and I generally felt down. I did what was on offer on the National Health: traction, including hanging with my hands in the stair well, physiotherapy exercises, ultrasound and deep heat treatment. Then, as that had little effect, osteopathy and chiropractic treatments, different kinds of massage, yoga, acupuncture and Tai Chi.

Perhaps the one thing I should not have chosen to do as a profession was dance. Having completed a drama and theatre arts course I found that words were less 'my thing' as a means of expression than movement. My back was less troublesome when moving about, which had the effect of masking the discomforts. In 1973 I went to the Laban Art of Movement Centre and enjoyed my time there enormously, doing the dance theatre course with a teacher who taught the Martha Graham Technique in my second year. My back problems did not improve and, as much as I loved the course, practising that technique with its rigour of contraction and release did not help my situation at all.

During my time at the Laban Centre I was introduced to the idea of the AT by my father. With the demand of dance practice, rehearsal and performance, I was suffering with back pain. I went to a teacher in Richmond, Surrey for a while, but found the lessons, though quite nice, not very informative. With the travel being time consuming and exams on the way, Alexander lessons were dropped. But a seed had been sown.

I went back to college in 1976 to qualify to teach drama. Teaching opportunities took off from there: in youth centres, after school dance and drama clubs, adult evening classes and a production of Oliver! for an amateur operatic society.

Discomfort and pain were still a problem. Although I had decided the demand of performance work would be too great to cope with, I nevertheless thought that I'd be OK if I could do a solo show. It was a different challenge, doing all the choreography myself with the aim of touring the West Midlands. My inspiration was to bring together original poetry and music composition with reciters and musicians, and to design stage set, dresses and costumes. Of course a team of people were involved in everything that goes into putting a show on the road.

Later I became involved with a trio of girls, 'Even Stevens'. We toured the West Midlands, giving performances and workshops in schools and to the general public. The inaugurator of this group, Jayne Stevens, who was having lessons, was my next contact with the Alexander Technique.

I was in a bad way when I first started having lessons with her teacher, (much later on, he said my back was one of the worst he'd seen). He was very encouraging and gave me a first real glimpse of hope. Within a relatively short time of having lessons, it was liberating not to experience pain and discomfort when walking down the road after a lesson. Within nine months, I joined the teachers' training course. I thought that if I could be helped in this way, then that was what I wanted to do for others. My teacher was the training course director, and he brought a tremendous richness and variety to learning what the Technique was all about and how to apply it in practice.

The Technique provided me with an answer to my back problem, but little did I realise the extent of a much slower process of learning to put into practice the central concept of the Technique of inhibiting habitual reactions. Our thinking on every level was challenged: how could it be otherwise when the very essence of how we use ourselves is the unity of mind and body? What we think affects muscle tension and therefore our posture. Recognising this is a continuous, ongoing process of developing awareness of how we think and react in all life's situations, and how to apply conscious, reasoned control to any activity, mind and body together. It is possible, for example, not to fly off the handle when provoked or to sit without rounding over while studying.

I could certainly relate to the idea of 'pulling down' as being that churning of the mind in having to make a difficult decision, assessing what might be right or wrong, dealing with a work load, or with the challenges of studying. The pain in my back and legs returned unmistakably in problematic situations. I learned how to recognise and inhibit unhelpful thought processes, and direct my thinking and activity so that the pain would eventually go away.

As I grew in understanding, the Technique became something that was not only to do with the wonderful supportive work at the hands of the teacher that helped to 'sort my back out', but also with identifying and understanding my own habitual reactions. I learned to reason things through with the view of wanting not to stiffen our necks nor to pull ourselves out of shape. F.M. Alexander said in *Man's Supreme Inheritance* that a changed point of view is the royal road to reformation. This was an approach that truly dealt with 'having to learn to live with it' to the point that I could relinquish the idea that I even had a bad back. I was learning how to apply myself to the very things I believed I could not do, and one of them was academic study. Good use is about maintaining good posture and efficiency of movement through conscious, reasoned thought.

I qualified in 1987 and moved to Stockton-on-Tees where I joined a colleague. Together, we built a private practice and ran courses between Newcastle-upon-Tyne and Darlington, and worked also with other colleagues in the North East at the time. When she moved on to pastures new in 1990, she encouraged me to take on her pupils in Stockton and Newcastle, and I continued with two other venues in Redcar and Durham as well. Three years later, my energy with working and travelling by public transport ran out. I had to relinquish Newcastle and Redcar. Since then I have continued in private practice in Stockton and Durham. It is the work I have found to be my vocation.

I met the man of my life in 1999 and we were married in 2004. My new family included a wonderful teenage stepson and a boisterous collie cross spaniel dog. Trying to control and retrain a dog was not easy, but at a certain stage I realised the true meaning of, 'if you can't change the external circumstances then change your attitude toward it'.

This continues to be a motto for change for me: if I can truly recognise whether the problem lies within me or in the external circumstance, the process of conscious inhibition and reasoned choices can begin in earnest in the direction of changing one's response. As F.M. Alexander said, 'My technique is based on inhibition, the inhibition of undesirable, unwanted responses to stimuli and hence it is primarily a technique for the development of the control of human reaction.' (*The Universal Constant in Living*, p. 88 )

I began a new journey when I joined an Alexander Technique teachers' organisation in 2007. I have enjoyed the support of a good friend and colleague, and the newness and opportunities of different continuing professional development (CPD) sessions on offer. Over the next two years my life changed: the pain in my back and legs was getting worse and I realised I could no longer sustain myself. Colleagues helped me greatly with hands-on work to assist in finding some resolve to the situation. Discussion ensued as to whether the situation in my back had in fact changed. A scan showed an increased slippage, and the possibility of an operation was researched and discussed.

All this took a great deal of deliberation, as I had to scrutinise my belief in myself and my ability to apply and teach the Technique, and whether it was a deterioration in my ability that had caused a worsening of the situation. It was a dark time of serious consideration. After all, I had been teaching for twenty years, so I should have been pretty good at it! I was reassured when I realised that even with the best use wear and tear with age is inevitable. Some people with spondylolisthesis can live a pain-free existence until they reach their fifties and problems can tend to begin then.

In August 2010 I had a five-hour operation to fuse the fourth lumbar vertebra to the sacrum, securing the fifth vertebra from any further movement. The AT is a wonderful tool pre- and post-operatively, and I thank my lucky stars that I am as good as I am, with no major pain in my back and legs, which I'd suffered before. There are other aches and pains of recovery to work through as nerve, muscle and bone continue to repair. I am hopeful of continued improvement for years to come yet. I cannot imagine how I would have managed and would continue to manage without applying the principles of the AT and the support of Christian friends, family and colleagues. I think I have been lucky in my life to have had the opportunity of learning the Alexander Technique, which saved me from an operation earlier in my life, and which has given me a whole new direction in life.

# The Way Back from Losing a Voice and a Career
## Keith Hawkins

My job as a solicitor involved a great deal of talking. Indeed, almost non-stop talking!

Some years ago I developed a cold which resulted in me losing my voice and then, after a particularly stressful day, my voice completely gave way. I was not particularly concerned. I believed that after a little rest all would be well. However, when it didn't come back I became worried, anxious and stressed. The longer it went on, the more it seemed to compound the problem: communicating with anyone – clients, staff and family – became more and more difficult. Ultimately I had to give up work on medical advice because the stress was damaging my health.

I sought medical advice, but nobody could find a physical cause. I consulted ENT specialists, neurologists, psychiatrists and psychologists. All were baffled. I then had speech therapy, which had little effect. During the course of the therapy I was referred to a plastic surgeon. Further investigations showed that I had ' a floppy soft palate' – probably resulting from viral damage at the time of the original infection. This caused the excessive nasal air loss during speech, which made communication so difficult. To try to overcome this problem, the surgeon injected Bio-Alcamid (a tissue filler usually used in cosmetic surgery) to try to stabilise the palate. This procedure was of minimal benefit and resulted in me having sleep apnoea and heavy snoring. I now have to use a respirator at night to help me breathe. I have been told this will gradually wear off as the effect of the injection wears off.

I was beginning to despair, until a friend of mine suggested that the Alexander Technique might help. As luck would have it I knew an AT teacher in my village who agreed to take me on. I have had regular lessons and have come to realise that, although the initial cause of the problem was probably physical, if I become anxious, stressed and frustrated it exacerbates the situation and my voice becomes more strangled and difficult to understand.

Gradually, through constant practice and attention to the Alexander Technique, my voice has improved considerably, to the point where I am generally understood – even on the telephone, which was a particular problem. Thus, my quality of life is much enhanced, and I am able to enjoy company and conversation that for the last five or six years has been impossible.

I do, however, have to be constantly vigilant. I am a rather excitable sort of chap and if I forget to pay attention my voice still 'goes pear-shaped'! I must remind myself to momentarily STOP talking, allow my breathing to normalise, relax my palate and use Alexander directions to regain my composure.

Thanks to my teacher and the AT I once again lead a full, happy, normal life.

# The Freedom to Ascend
## Jennet Blake

I cannot remember where I heard about the Alexander Technique, but my first real encounter was very dramatic. Attending a Saturday morning course, I learnt the AT art of walking upstairs and how to carry parcels and bags. As I had been hauling myself upstairs by the banisters, it was a revelation to discover that I had the freedom to ascend without any external help. Twenty years later, at eighty-one, I can still climb stairs without assistance and know how to carry weights and stay in balance (even if many things are now too heavy to carry!).

Overjoyed with success, I attended a week's holiday course, which proved to be the ideal way of learning to live an Alexander life without distraction. The overall effect lasted for many weeks. One or two further courses reinforced much of what I had learnt as well as opening new areas. An 'extra three inches' was added to my height so that I regained the height I had had at twenty-one, and which I appear to still retain. At work, the AT gave me extra confidence, and I felt as tall as others who were often, in reality, taller than me. I could only wish that I had learnt the Technique much earlier in my life.

Over several years, as I retired and moved around, I went to a number of teachers, all of whom helped me in various ways. One helped to straighten out the scoliosis in my back. I encouraged my horse-riding daughter to see her and she realised how much AT could contribute to the teaching of riding. Eventually my daughter trained as a teacher and now she teaches both riding and AT.

I am aware that I am not a 'good' AT student because I am very forgetful and find it hard to remember to inhibit and to lie down every day. However, I am absolutely convinced that it has transformed my life and allowed me to be active in playing croquet, gardening, driving my car and looking after small grandchildren, all of which are fundamental parts of my life.

# Never Too Old to Start
Thomas Newton

Let me introduce myself to give you a picture of who I am, and how and why I came to be involved with the Alexander Technique. I am Thomas Derek Newton, married, eighty-one years old (never too old to start the Alexander Technique, as I have learned), five foot, six inches tall and weighing just under ten stone, which is about the same weight as when I left the parachute regiment aged twenty-three, after my two years of National Service in 1951–53. I am fortunate to have good health except for my back problem which began in my mid-thirties while teaching carpentry and joinery. I was moving a sheet of nineteen mm blockboard measuring eight foot by four foot with a student who let go of his end in a gust of wind. I tried to hold it, and out went my back. From then on my back has given me trouble from time to time, until, in my mid-seventies it became chronic, sometimes with acute pain. This in turn changed my life.

'What if' took over. I had been windsurfing for a number of years; 'what if' my back gave out? How would I get back to shore? I felt for my wife's sake and my own safety I would have to give up windsurfing. I thought walking might help: many articles recommended walking as a gentle exercise, but not in my case. One morning, about one and a half miles from home, the pain made me cry out. I was immobile for a few minutes; my back had 'gone out'. I managed painfully to struggle home.

I decided to seek advice from my doctor, who sent me for an X-ray. The findings were:

> There is a narrowing of L3/L4, L5/S1 intervertebral disc space.

I was told that this meant that two of my lower vertebrae were compressed. What could I do, I asked my GP? He said I could try physiotherapy, but wasn't sure how long it might take to be referred. Chiropractor? Worth a try, he said. It did help but was not long lasting, sometimes for a few days or a week. Then, I suppose, I went back to my old habits of doing things badly. The various exercises I have always done to keep me supple and fit did not help my back. I spent a lot of time and money trying to find something that would help my back, without taking pills.

We threw out our old three-piece suite and bought another, gave that away to our daughter and bought our current one. A 'memory' twin mattress was another buy, still in use. We changed our car because the current one has a more suitable seat for long journeys. I read a number of articles and books on back problems. If you suffer from a bad back, I feel sure that, like me, you would try almost anything.

A medical examination revealed that I have Paget's disease. The lower part of my left leg has thickened and is bent forward. There is no cure for Paget's. The thickened and bent leg has been with me for many years and does not incapacitate me. I had thought the bend was due to the weight I put on it when flat-green bowling. My action when delivering the bowl is to put my left elbow on my left knee. This puts almost all my body weight onto my leg. Thirty years of doing this made me think that the way I bowled had done the damage. It turned out to be Paget's disease.

Why do I have to bowl with the elbow on the knee and give up windsurfing? In my early apprentice days as a carpenter and joiner I developed arthritic knees. Nobody told me to use knee pads or a kneeler when nailing floorboards for days. At seventeen years old, I had never heard of housemaid's knee, where the knees swell up, and in my case end up arthritic. In the 1940s, Health and Safety had not been thought of. This early injury to my knees helped stop me windsurfing in my mid-seventies because my damaged knees would not allow me to waterstart. The wind in the sail picks you up out of the water, which requires effort through the knees. I had to rely on pulling the sail out of the water, against the wind and with water in the sail, which requires a lot of effort in the arms and back. When my back problem became chronic, I had to give up board sailing for safety reasons and because of my wife's concern for my welfare on the sea. I knew it worried her.

I suppose it is reasonable to assume that an injury at seventeen may have led to back trouble at seventy-one, and being unable to lift using my knees.

My Alexander Technique teacher and myself belong to a small art group who hire a village hall for our evening session. This means moving tables and chairs at the beginning and end of the evening. Even though I was having back problems, I was helping to move the furniture. It was apparent to the AT teacher that I had a back problem. Twice she offered me advice on how to stand and have my body and head properly balanced. This was not an Alexander lesson, but a few minutes of kind advice. The name Alexander Technique stuck in my mind. A fairly large book with an equally long title, *The Complete Illustrated Encyclopaedia of Alternative Healing Therapies*, carried an eight-page article with illustrations. This gave a good description of Alexander and the Technique. Another member of our art group told me she was having Alexander lessons, with this teacher. About the same time, a doctor was giving a talk to the patient participation group at our local surgery on research he was doing. During the talk he asked if anyone had heard of the Alexander Technique. He went on to describe it and said that he followed its teachings. One thing after another kept cropping up about the Alexander Technique, enough for me to ask the teacher if she would take me, even at my age, as a pupil, and it all began. To me another life-changing experience.

Through the lessons I have had, the number of things I can do is remarkable, compared to how it was previously. My back is not completely cured, but has become easily managed. No longer is there a debilitating ache with a feeling it could 'go out' at any time.

My outlook on life and my physical ability have, without doubt, radically changed since starting the Alexander Technique under the tuition of my great teacher, whose method is exactly how I like it to be.

We need a teacher for the same reason that even top sports people need a coach or adviser. Watch any golf tournament or snooker player on television, and the commentators can see what is wrong with a golfer's swing, or what the snooker player's action or mental attitude is. It is often slowed down so that we can also see what they mean. Often these actions have become a habit which is hard to break.

One of my pastimes is indoor flat-green bowling. A session of bowls last two hours. To play the game requires a fair amount of bending to deliver the bowl a few inches from the ground, standing at the head (where the bowls come to rest), walking to and fro at each end. During the onset of my back problem I sometimes had difficulty bowling, either getting into a position to deliver the bowl, or in standing for any length of time. Since starting the Alexander Technique, these difficulties are no longer present.

My working life began at the age of sixteen, after two years on a pre-apprenticeship course at my local technical college. At twenty-one, I did two years' National Service in the parachute regiment. After National Service I worked as a carpenter and joiner for eleven years. Looking back, this was physically hard work, and at that time most work was done by hand. Lorries were unloaded by hand; now one man can unload using machinery. Cement came in bags weighing 112 pounds. Even as an apprentice, I was expected to carry them. Other jobs stopped to unload the lorry quickly if it was raining. Now cement comes in bags weighing only fifty-six pounds.

Retiring from teaching carpentry and joinery at a technical college about sixteen years ago, I have continued to do gardening, home maintenance and other building work.

Our daughter convinced us to take out our bath, the side of which we had to step over after showering. Being an occupational therapist and more experienced than my wife or myself in the matter of getting older, a wet room with shower was decided on. We got a plumber and tiler to do the finishing. I was to take off the old tiles. As our house is a fairly modern bungalow, the walls of the bathroom were tiled onto a plasterboard studwork wall. The tiles were well stuck. It was no easy task getting them off, and some of the plasterboard got badly damaged, while other parts had tile adhesive firmly stuck. Lining all the walls with half-inch (13mm) thick marine plywood seemed the solution to getting a straight surface for the new tiles. As well, the holes and old adhesive would be covered. I decided, due to successfully managing my problem back, I could do the job. The work involved heaving and cutting large, awkward, heavy sheets of plywood and getting them on to benches for cutting and drilling. The sort of work I had done fifty years before while teaching.

'Give it some thought, how could I apply the Alexander way to it? What is the easiest way? What has my teacher told me to do? Stop, think. Don't set off into my old habit of just getting on with it.'

The first thing I did was to decide on the amount of time to be spent working. 'Use a kitchen timer set at three quarters of an hour, never more than an hour. Do not jump back to the usual habit of, "I will just finish this bit". Stop, sit down and do Alexander Technique of sitting in a chair, relaxing. Set the timer to fifteen minutes resting.'

Working in this pattern, with up to one and a half hour long meal breaks, work could carry on until well into the evening.

What my teacher has taught me is to stop and think. This, for me, is a hard thing to do. I wrote this down after my first lesson, 'How will I remember to stop and think, visualise what I am about to do?'

The great thing about the Alexander way is being able to do it anytime, anywhere: nobody knows you are practising it. All you need is a teacher (a sort of coach). I know I have got a brilliant one. The difference between standing with weight on one leg more than the other and being in balance is not noticeable in a queue of people. Getting up from a sitting position using Alexander Technique does not appear to be that much different to a casual observer, but the difference is immense. No longer do I leap out of a chair thinking 'I will just do…' This is an old habit which I am still trying to break, along with many others acquired over many years. This is, for me, the hard part.

The easiest way to hurt my back is to lean partially forward – say to clean the far side of the bath. 'My back feels alright, it won't take a minute. I'll risk it'.

Stop, think about it, weeks, days may be required to get the back better again. Stop, think, kneel down, lean onto the near side, clean the part in front of you, then move across to a new position left or right, do not stretch. This sounds so easy, but the temptation is not to get something to kneel on, to stretch a bit too far, to resort to my lifetime habit of 'I will just do…' Stretch too far, lift too much, stay in one position too long, especially when working at my bench. Now I am trying to develop a new habit of 'Not just do…'

It is impossible to turn the clock back. I know that at eighty, I cannot do the things which were easy at twenty. What I decided, and told my Alexander teacher I would do, was to get the best possible use out of my body, which is all anyone can do and, being lucky enough to find a good teacher and give my all to the Alexander Technique, I am able to do things that I would have considered impossible seven months ago.

Something else worth mentioning: between lessons nineteen and twenty, while delivering plants to my daughter's house, I got out of the car and walked up a slope, up a few steps and on to what was to be a patio area. My son-in-law was getting the foundations straight and to a fall ready for slate slabs. He had got a lot of the work done but I could see the struggle he was having getting it straight and to a fall. We work well together: he is an office worker, but a keen DIY enthusiast and is always ready to take advice. We set to, getting things straight and, even though I was not dressed for the occasion, worked for thirty to forty-five minutes, shovelling, raking and barrowing.

When I got back in the car to go home I thought, 'I never once thought about my back'. Looking back as I write now, before taking up the Alexander Technique I could barely walk up the slope to their house without back pain. I would not have even thought of getting on with the physical work. My daughter has stopped telling my wife that I am walking badly as I go up to their house. Thinking about it, I probably sit better and drive better, and use the Alexander Technique to get out of the car before walking up the slope and steps.

# The Emerging Self
Jane Evans

I was drifting in and out of consciousness as the (wonderful) firemen were cutting me out of the tangled wreckage of our car; I remember apologising for being a nuisance and wondering if I'd make it to my son's graduation the following month. I was in the front passenger seat of our Montego Estate car. A big Volvo had come out at a junction straight into me, and knocked our car sideways into the oncoming traffic. I'd taken another bashing, this time from a large Saab. All three cars were wrecked, but fortunately I was the only one really badly injured.

The scar on my head still gives a Harry Potter tingle occasionally, but the bones and soft tissues have healed amazingly and very few people pick up on the asymmetry caused by breaking my pelvis. (I'm so grateful for the consultant in one of my follow-up visits saying that I'd be back to normal in about six months – and then coming back to say that 'normal' didn't mean the same as before the accident.)

I've always been afraid of having a car crash, but although I wouldn't want to go through it again, or wish it on anybody, the overall experience was an incredibly positive one for me. When I came home from hospital I was amazed at the wonder of being alive, by the green of the trees against the blue of the sky, the white of the clouds, the birdsong, the love and joy that enfolded me; and the wonder of the healing process, my whole being programmed to regenerate itself; the daily, weekly, monthly alterations; the realisation that, somehow, all was well. All of life ahead was bonus time. A lot of what I believed seemed somehow to have made that long, long journey from head to heart. (I had often told people wholeheartedly that their value didn't depend on their usefulness – now I began to grasp that my own didn't either!)

Two of my daughters, who'd had Alexander Technique lessons in music college, suggested that lessons would help me. The insurance company agreed to pay for twenty lessons. I had no idea what I was letting myself in for!

My husband was a vicar (retired now), and twelve years older than me. We'd had seven children, including two sets of twins, in eight years; life in a vicarage is as rich and full as anyone could want (often more so). I'd never been in paid employment, and a clergy stipend was such that it allowed for the faith that God will provide to become deep-rooted. To have money to spend on the 'luxury' of the Alexander Technique was a challenge to me; surely this money could be put to better use, I thought.

I'd read a bit about the Technique (I've always liked to be 'prepared' and 'in charge') and I was mystified, but open to learn. I expected to learn to 'use myself better' in the sense of being more poised and efficient.

Initially, I thought I was paying for moon shine, or the 'emperor's new clothes'. I'd read chemistry and maths at university and liked to make rational sense of things; I liked to do well at whatever I undertook. With the Alexander Technique I found I could do neither! In a very pleasant but nebulous way I felt 'lighter' and 'taller' but if it hadn't been for my husband encouraging me, and if it wasn't for the fact that the lessons were being paid for, I'm sure I would have stopped; I am so glad I persevered.

I would echo John Dewey's words, which he used in his preface to one of Alexander's books:

> *In bringing to bear whatever knowledge I already possessed – or thought I did – and whatever powers of discipline I had acquired... I had the most humiliating experience of my life, intellectually speaking. For to find that one is unable to execute directions, including inhibitory ones, in doing such a seemingly simple act as to sit down, when one is using all the mental capacity which one prides himself upon possessing, is not an experience congenial to one's vanity ... I found the things that I had 'known' – in the sense of theoretical belief –... changed into vital experiences which gave a new meaning to the knowledge of them. (The Use of the Self, 1932, p. 10)*

I began to be aware that a lot was happening, (even if I didn't seem to be 'doing' anything) if I stopped trying to 'get it right' and 'allowed' myself to not react to a stimulus in a habitual way. I liked this feeling of 'lightness' and was reminded of G.K. Chesterton's 'Angels can fly because they take themselves lightly'. I was amazed one day on the way home by train from the 'Good Food Show' taking my heavy rucksack off and feeling myself, very unexpectedly, spring up! As Frank Pierce-Jones says:

> *Once I had experienced the kinaesthetic effect, the reward was so great that I tried to recapture it directly and to hang on to it when I had it. This proved self-defeating, however. It was the indirect effect of a psycho-physical process and could only be obtained by not trying for it.... Inhibition is a negative term but it describes a positive process... The immediate effect of Alexandrian inhibition is a sense of freedom, as if a heavy garment has been removed. (Jones, Freedom to Change, p. 10–11)*

I realised that my Alexander Technique lessons were having a big impact on every aspect of my life and at this point (about six months after my lessons started and after I'd had about fifteen lessons) I started to keep a journal of notes and quotes and pictures about my Alexander experience, my own words on the left-hand page and pictures and quotations on the right. I've never been a journal-keeper, but this one continued and I treasure it as being full of pictorial and verbal and poetic images of my voyage of discovery, and sometimes quite a source of amusement at myself.

I titled it *The Emerging Self* – which seemed right at the time! The trouble is that words cannot adequately describe or explain experience; as Alexander himself said, 'Be careful of the printed matter: you may not read it as it is written down.' What I've written and quoted, and the pictures I've stuck in my book can act as triggers for me, but they may evoke something completely different for you! 'I know you believe you understand what you think I said, but what I want you to realise is that what you heard is not what I meant.' (Strangely enough, I reached the back cover of the book at the same time as my last lesson before I started training as an AT teacher). What follows is a selection of 'snapshots', an incomplete and potentially misleading account of isolated – but linked – events in my Alexander journey!

I called the first 'chapter' of my journal 'Farewell to Shadowlands' and quoted C.S. Lewis from *The Last Battle*:

...Do you remember? Do you remember?...

...Dare we? Is it right?...

...Can it be meant for us?

I then continued with what I remembered of my initial impressions; my expectations and my experience. At the start of the journal I wrote that:

I learned to stand, sit, walk, go up and down stairs, to breathe – or rather I was shown and taught to – or rather I unlearned some of my habitual ways of doing things (and a new way is starting to emerge). A lot of this is conveyed by touch as well as verbal instructions, hands being used to clarify and reinforce verbal messages.

It was so difficult to articulate what Alexander Technique is and does!

For part of each lesson I lay on an Alexander table. I perceived the Alexander 'table' as the doctor's examination couch – experienced mostly during pregnancy and after our car crash – or the delivery bed – the place where my babies came into the world. So the AT table, for me, had connotations of the place where I was totally exposed and vulnerable. But where something life-changing and miraculous (even if somewhat painful) could happen. The place where my innermost recesses were probed. The place where I met with life and death.

And this exposed me to myself, and enlarged and expanded me so that I could no longer fit in my familiar – if dark, damp, and cramped – 'cave' (even if I wanted to).

F.M. says, 'There is no disrobing.' But there was for me a huge exposure, which I found very scary at times. We talk glibly about being 'in touch' or 'in contact' with people, but actually, bodily, we hardly ever are except with those we're intimate with. Also, we have, in my opinion, so sexualised our idea of touch that we've become 'out of touch' with ourselves and others – to our great loss. I was very blessed in my home and marriage relationships but even so I felt somewhat embarrassed(?), confused(?), unsure(?) about lying on a bed(?) while my teacher put hands on me and somehow moved bits of me about – all the more so because I enjoyed it!

There was no sense of anything inappropriate, but it was just so unfamiliar, somewhat surreal, and I wasn't sure what the boundaries were, if there were any, or if boundaries were appropriate anyway; I was out of my 'comfort-zone'. The touch was so 'releasing' and felt so good and seemed to be reaching so deep inside my being that I was almost afraid of the whole process; I somehow found it hard to feel that it was alright to feel so good – I think I would have found it easier if I'd had to make a big effort, to do something, not just stop and think these things called 'directions'!

There was also such a sense of wholeness and homecoming to it all; my whole being was involved; I couldn't make much sense of what was happening, not just in my body but in my whole being, but I somehow knew that it was good; I was eating from the 'tree of life'. In terms of awareness of undue tension, it reminded me of the relaxation and breathing methods that I'd used so effectively that I had needed no analgesia when I was giving birth to my children.

Before I had AT lessons, I was beginning to think I was past my 'best-before'; now I knew that 'the best is yet to be'. To say that my lessons were the high points of my month might give the impression that my life was dull; on the contrary, everything I already enjoyed became so much more fun. Sometimes I felt I could hardly contain the life in me – as if it was bursting out of me, as if I was somehow incandescent. Everything seemed richer and fuller, more 'colourful' – and easier. It was as if everything was falling naturally into place and flowing well. I felt in love with life.

*Inhibition*

All this was an exhilarating, scary voyage of discovery. I don't have the language to articulate what happened; the only words I have are either mystical or erotic (and maybe that's why lots of mystical experiences are described in erotic language), as if the whole experience had a similar 'fullness' to worship or love-making though it was neither; a fullness of life and living. And although it was unfamiliar, it fitted well with my experience of God's sense of humour in his dealings with me!

In my lessons I was safely taken beyond and outside all the boundaries I knew I had, and many that I wasn't aware of. I realised I was 'exploring my edges', as it were; taken to the edge of a cliff, being gently pushed, finding myself flying. My body feeling so spacious. It was a wonderful experience and caused me a lot of 'self-discovery'!! I knew then that going forward would cost 'not less than everything (a condition of complete simplicity')– to misquote T.S. Eliot (*Four Quartets*), and that total openness to the 'process'/'journey/'adventure' was my only real option if I wanted to really and truly look at AT – and at myself; a big challenge. Michelangelo was once asked why he was struggling with a block of stone and replied, 'because there's an angel in there and I want to set him free.' I'd experienced this liberation in my so-called 'spiritual' life; now I was discovering it through the whole of me, all of who I am, my being, body, mind, spirit and every other labelled 'bit', altogether, in unity.

My journal at this stage was full of quotes and pictures; T.S. Eliot was, as always, inspirational, and Piet Hein's pithy *Grooks* perceptive and amusing. I remember one of my daughters saying, 'Mum, do you have to sit up straight like that all the time?' It came as a shock – and a great deal of excitement – to me that I was, quite effortlessly, sitting up straight, that this AT stuff was working for me in a way that was visible to my family!

I have another entry noting that I'd grown taller. I'd noticed that things on a shelf were unfamiliarly at my eye-level and found I had 'grown' over an inch. But as well as physical height growth, I feel as if I've expanded, become more who I am, more free to be who I am.

It doesn't make, or try to make, me something that I'm not, but it calls me forth, it helps me to emerge, to be more me, more who I am.

I wrote, *If I discover/uncover/realise who I AM, is that God in me?*

I preached AT ad nauseam with the zeal of the convert to my long-suffering family and friends and anyone else who'd listen, and I read nothing but AT books!

It was at around the time I'd had about twenty lessons I started to know that I wanted to teach, that I was in this for good, for good and for ever; but at that point the three-year full-time training seemed an impossible dream. I called the next chapter: 'Further Up and Further In', again inspired by C.S. Lewis's *The Last Battle*.

> *It was only a shadow or a copy of the real Narnia which has always been here and always will be here. And of course it's different; as different as a real thing is from a shadow or as waking life is from a dream.'... It was the unicorn who summed up what everyone was feeling, 'I belong here. This is the land I have been looking for all my life, though I never knew till now.'*

I felt like a seed, bursting and coming out into the – scary – daylight, or a caterpillar undergoing all the unfamiliar stages of change into butterfly. I learnt to do 'nothing' and to be still in the waiting, 'pregnant' plateaux times when nothing seemed to change and the euphoria calmed down too. I altered shape and size and grew up. I read a book by Walter Carrington. In the introduction it mentioned when he was born and I realised his ninetieth birthday was coming up. I decided to make him a birthday card, and sent it off with a letter thanking him for all the help the book had been to me. I was very surprised and delighted to receive a reply and an invitation to have a lesson with him! I made the expedition to London and had a wonderful meeting with him – and he didn't even charge me for the lesson, which turned out to be one of the last ones he gave before he died. I was so blessed.

I wrote just before my journal ended:

The 'best' bits so far?
- The whole terrifying, exciting journey.
- Clearing out so much clutter, and unearthing so many treasures in the process.
- Having so much fun.
- Coming out of a prison I didn't know I was in.
- Finding more colours in the rainbow.
- Hearing the tune, not just the words.
- 'Falling in love', becoming a child again, and growing up.

And the 'worst' bits?
- Being an archetypal end-gainer!
- The plateaux.
- Feeling discouraged.
- Confronting all my insecurities (over and over again)!
- Not knowing if I was going to fly or fall when I was in mid-air.

But the best and worst bits are only two sides of the same coin, really. Many things have made that longest of journeys from head to heart. I now know things I already knew, and I'm learning all the time.

It's the end of the beginning.

All that I've written is just the tip of the iceberg – there's so much more.

I finished the journal with the words my lessons used to end with: That's enough for today.

## Unreliable Sensory Appreciation

> *For the time being the child's body was comparatively straightened out, that is, without the extreme twists and distortions that had been so noticeable when she came into the room. When this was done, the little girl looked across at her mother and said to her in an indescribable tone, 'Oh! Mummie, he's pulled me out of shape.'*
> *(Constructive Conscious Control, p. 94)*

> *He must recognize that guidance by his old sensory appreciation (feeling) is dangerously faulty, and he must be taught to regain his lost power of inhibition and to develop conscious guidance.*
> *(Constructive Conscious Control, p. 43–44)*

Some indication of the role of unreliable sensory appreciation has already been given in the section on *Recognition of the Force of Habit*. (See page 21.) Indeed the first quotation in this section indicates further the interconnectedness of Alexander's concepts relating it to inhibition. *Unreliable sensory appreciation* includes sensory experiences conveyed through all the senses, in particular the kinaesthetic sense, which are the triggers for psycho-physical action and reaction.

As long as we have not acquired a clear idea of 'what is required for the successful performance of a certain act', together with 'a knowledge of the psycho-physical means whereby those requirements can be met', the mode of control we choose is likely to be haphazard. What if our success is due to chance or good luck? Can we ever be certain of repeating it? In the long run, Alexander argues, an approach based on the trial-and-error method and unreliable sensory appreciation contributes considerably to diminishing our chances of succeeding; and repeated errors are bound to reinforce the uncertainty and fear.

Alison Franks rejects a course of steroid injections for back pain because, she says, 'I need the pain to know what the hell I'm doing, because I know how badly behaved I can be if I feel fine.' But the question follows: once you recognise how badly you behave, how do you go about changing that behaviour?

Christine Green reaches the realisation that it is 'time to give up a habit I'd had for over thirty years of sitting on a cushion when I was driving. I had convinced myself that I couldn't drive without it. I took a chance, and I was quite safe!'

Richard Brennan cannot see what his Alexander Technique teacher is talking about until the teacher 'placed a mirror in front of me and I could clearly see that I was twisting to the right while leaning at least twenty degrees to the left. Yet, despite the fact that I could clearly see that I was sitting in a very crooked way, I still "felt" perfectly straight.'

Acknowledging that you cannot rely on how things feel – on your sensory appreciation, which has accumulated over a lifetime – is a big step toward allowing the possibility of change.

# Forward and Up at Seventy-Five
Roey Burden

I have had to learn to walk six times during my life, if you count the very first time as a rather plump toddler!

In 1935, when I was three years old, my mother noticed both my knees and my left ankle were swollen. The doctors decided hospital and bed rest were the answer and I was admitted to the South London Hospital for Women. As to what treatment, if any, I received, no one remembers, but I suppose it worked. I was sent home after nine months and learnt to walk, as an even-plumper toddler, for the second time.

At the age of ten, the same swelling occurred and, once again, the answer was hospital, where I was diagnosed with juvenile rheumatoid arthritis (Still's disease). I was not allowed to put any weight on my legs, so was confined to bed and given gold injections once a week with a vast needle and syringe wielded by one nurse whilst another held me down. They were very, very painful. I became very allergic to the gold, which had the effect of covering me with a rash. So eventually they were stopped. Heat treatment followed, and I can remember the agony of having a cage of burning electric light bulbs put over my knees and being unable to move away from the intense heat until a nurse came to turn it off.

At that time no one disputed a doctor's verdict, but I do now, and am convinced their diagnosis was made as some sort of 'label' which had to be attached to my notes. Still's disease causes pain and deformities – I had neither. However, after nearly a year I was sent home, having learnt to walk again for the third time.

Thirteen years old and off we go to hospital (Great Ormond Street) once more – both knees and left ankle swollen, but no pain, no stiffness, so same diagnosis. This time the treatment was slightly bizarre, as apart from the obligatory bed rest, large wads of cotton wool soaked in liquid paraffin were wrapped round my knees every night and bandaged up tightly. No physiotherapy was given. I was there for nearly a year before I was sent home in a wheelchair. After some weeks, the GP said I could walk again and go back to school. He took one arm, my father the other, and that was the fourth time. No walking frame, no crutches, no stick – just working it out for myself with the aid of anything I could hold on to.

Some twenty years on, after our second daughter was born in 1963, both knees suddenly became swollen again – the ankle had dropped out of contention by this time. The doctors tried steroid injections and withdrawing the fluid from my knee (over a pint came out), but neither worked for any length of time, so they decided the answer was an operation called a synovectomy (removal of the synovial tissue). My right knee, being the worst of the two offenders, was duly operated on, although they were intending to do both together. But I had found a voice (albeit rather small) of protest by then and refused.

I was told I would be three weeks in hospital, but should have known better than to believe that. The operation involved cutting through nerves and muscle. This time physiotherapists were standing by the bed telling me to lift my leg before I had even come round from the anaesthetic! The size and weight of the bandage alone was enough to make this nearly impossible – and, for me, it was. Despite physio three times a day, it took me three weeks to achieve a slight lift and then only by looking to my left. Finally, after nine weeks, I managed a few steps aided by a walking frame and two physios.

I was walking again for the fifth time, but the legacy of the operation was a tendency for the right foot to kick out by itself uncontrollably, particularly when going downstairs. After several near falls, I took to going down backwards (on the advice of a lighthouse keeper who was used to near-vertical steps) wherever I was – I got some funny stares, but took the view it was better to be safe and odd than sorry!

All remained the same for the next three decades. But then, I started tripping and catching with my right foot, and realised I was not picking it up correctly. A diagnosis of a dropped ankle was given by the consultant, and I was recommended for physiotherapy and an NHS ankle support. This turned out to be heavy, white plaster moulded from the back of my calf under my foot to the toes. I found it virtually impossible to walk in – apart from the blisters caused – so abandoned it. A CT scan followed, but revealed nothing. Nerve tests also came back with a negative verdict. The leading company in prosthetics did not think it was a dropped ankle and provided me with a support, fitted and moulded in plastic. This did help a bit, but I was still liable to trip, especially when tired, and my walking was getting more and more laboured due to my fear of falling. I was becoming limited as to where I could go without a car, and was offered a disabled parking permit.

One doctor gave me a reasonable explanation by saying that the nerves had obviously been cut during the operation and had not healed as they should, so were constantly trying to find where they should go and what they should do. Therefore, some days they were sending the correct messages to the brain and other days not. This made sense to me, but still did not provide a solution. I was having physiotherapy on a twice weekly basis as, by this time, my lower back was painful and felt 'stuck down'. The treatment and exercises always relieved the ache, but it would come back a few days later.

I had done yoga for some time, which helped keep my muscles active and did a lot for my morale and general wellbeing. At least that was something positive to look forward to every week. On the advice of the physio, I tried Pilates and stuck with it for two years, but it did not provide the answer.

About fifteen years earlier, I had attended an adult education class on the Alexander Technique, which was for six lessons only. We started off with nearly twenty pupils but by the second lesson this had dropped to eight. However, this gave the teacher an opportunity to give us all what I now know is called 'a turn'. I can clearly remember floating down the road afterwards. Why, oh, why did I not ask or look for more lessons then?

But my miracle was about to start: I met an Alexander Technique teacher who had just set up a centre for the Alexander Technique. From the very first lesson I felt different – a wonderful lightness that I remembered from before and a feeling of mental contentment as well.

After a month of weekly lessons, I became even more convinced this might be the answer, and so tried a week of lessons every day, and became totally convinced this was it, this was what I had been searching for. It did not happen overnight, but all my lessons helped and some produced 'Eureka moments'! How well I remember the first time I stood up from the chair without knowing how I got there, and how I would love that to happen again, but have to inhibit to stop end-gaining. Turns on the saddle were of enormous benefit – so much so that I bought a saddle chair to use at home when on the computer. This avoids what I call 'computer crouch'. An expensive purchase, but worth every penny (and it looks good too).

After the knee operation in 1964, I was told not to kneel again as, with no nerves in my knee, I could inadvertently kneel on a pin or nail. Although I cannot sit on my heels, I am not far off now through learning how to use my directions. Squatting was something not dreamt of, but again I can now do it – I often think of the photo of F.M. doing this – anything he could do, I can and will!

I enjoy the equipment which the teachers use to demonstrate the principles of the Technique: the trampoline, the balance board, juggling balls and scarves. Reading diaries written by past pupils are also of great help when you see they went through the same thinking of 'It's not possible' but then suddenly it is, and becomes second nature. Some DVDs of Walter Carrington teaching are also very helpful.

It was interesting to read of the experiences of a pupil of Alexander's, Carla Atkinson, from 1943. The following extract is remarkably similar to my own experiences:

> *The first noticeable change was that I was walking much better, not tiring so quickly and stepping off with more ease and lightness. I improved steadily and found that many little things I had been positive I could not do, I was doing. A surprising change was gradually taking place. As the so-called 'physical' change took place, a 'mental' change had to take place too, for we are all of*

*one piece. I found that I was up against all the destructive forces in myself and had to face and fight myself every moment. Thus, for the first time I really came to 'know' myself and to cease to be sorry for myself. Anyone who has been through such a training must have a clearer outlook on life and is, therefore, better fitted than heretofore to cope with whatever difficulties may be in store for him. It is hard for a person who has not experienced the release from physical tension given by this Technique to realise that wherever there is physical strain, there must be mental strain as well; that as soon as we are able consciously to give the directions which free the physical side of us, the mental side is relieved of tension and is thus able to function with greater clarity and ease. (Conscious Control, p. 28)*

Three years on now, and my life has been transformed. Finally, having learnt to walk for the sixth time, I am walking correctly. I had become so scared of falling I was walking with my shoulders held up in a rigid position. I constantly had my neck bent as I was looking down for any possible obstacles. My asthma was bad because my breathing was restricted, my pelvis likewise, and my legs only moved from the knees in small steps. Now my shoulders are relaxed, I can walk without looking down, just using my peripheral vision. My asthma is virtually gone and my 'Whispered Ah' deals with any breathing problems. My hips swinging, my legs striding out, I can walk without effort. I am floating and love every minute of my lessons, which have enabled me to be free to walk again where and when I want.

Of course, there have been various points that have proved more difficult than others. Relaxing the pelvis still is as, having walked incorrectly for years, my habit is to hold it up and back, which it still clings to. But at least I now know how it should not feel and am able to think it to the correct place. Releasing my ankles is another sticking point, but in one lesson my left ankle suddenly released taking both pupil and teacher by surprise, it was so dramatic! Another sticking point is keeping my feet evenly on the ground, when the right one in particular has a tendency to roll out, pulling the knees with it and tightening the inside of the thighs. But we are getting there by different ways of thinking. I have had to realise that the Alexander Technique is an ongoing way of living: there is no short cut and no certificate is ever awarded, as none of us will ever be perfect all of the time, but can only hope to be some of the time.

I have been immensely lucky in living near an Alexander Technique centre, and having available so many wonderful teachers who have all helped more than I can say. Lessons are such fun I cannot get enough of them and could be, and probably am, considered by some as an 'AT addict'! I introduced my eldest grandson to the centre and, apart from having lessons, he practises lying down every day, which he is convinced helped him through recent exams. He has definitely joined me as an 'addict'. My one sadness is that I did not discover the Alexander Technique years and years ago.

# Noticing Myself
## Christine Green

I found my way to Alexander lessons after reading a book in the library. It touched on the whole mind/body relationship and I immediately thought, 'Wow, I want some of this'. I had previously had a few non-specific joint pains and a doctor had told me that there was nothing wrong with me, to go away and stop thinking about it. I was also feeling a kind of emptiness in my life. I began to wonder about this and questioned exactly what I was doing to myself. Opening that book was the start for me.

My first contact with lessons was through a six week evening course, and I immediately had a feeling of new confidence that I could do things that before I had felt afraid to do or thought I couldn't do. Lying down every day seemed to release me from my usual way of thinking. I found I really enjoyed the suggested reading, whereas I had not really read many books since I had left school over thirty years earlier. School for me was learning, remembering and then repeating the information in an exam. It just had to be done, and I did it. I did as I was told and didn't seem to be able to act outside those rules and think for myself. I didn't do anything for myself.

I felt different about everything. For what seemed the first time in ages, I felt excited. This really meant something to me and I wanted to go on with it. I remember feeling great, but at the same time overwhelmed and when, after a few weeks, small setbacks happened I seemed to revert to letting all the doubts and fears come back into my life. I couldn't seem to find the feeling I'd had right at the beginning. Things were upsetting me again, and after about only half a dozen individual lessons I decided to stop. Even at this stage, I knew I would go back to Alexander, but it seemed not to be the right time for me.

I continued to think about the Alexander Technique on and off for the next four years, and then decided I would find another teacher. Even this was difficult for me to do. I had to find a name, make the phone call – I continually put it off: tomorrow, next week, another month, but all the time knowing I would do it. I had seen a different way of being. I realised that I didn't have to stay the way I was, and that I could make a choice and change things.

During the next set of lessons I found myself trying to find the same emotions and experiences I had previously had (I know now this is not possible). I kept a diary of what happened after each lesson and reading it recently helped me remember things I had forgotten. I stopped waking up with my heart thumping. For the first time in ages I slept through the night, my breathing felt easy, and one week I had written that my chest felt 'see through' – a really strange description but it was exactly how it felt. I seemed to fill the car seat after a lesson and I found myself smiling a lot more.

Other times I was cross with myself because of things I felt I was doing wrong. Changes were slower, I was impatient and sometimes nothing seemed to be happening. I nearly gave up but knew I couldn't. I gave up writing in my diary after three months because it seemed pointless and negative, but I still went to the lessons. I was still in a perpetual cycle of negative thinking. It had taken me over ten years to recognise this. I could see what I was doing and the circle just came round again and again. I knew it had to stop, but I didn't know how. It was as if my senses were deadened to everything around me because I was so concerned about myself.

Lying down was sometimes a struggle, as so many thoughts crowded into my head, distracting me constantly. A suggestion on how to deal with this worked so easily it surprised me. I thought it would be difficult but it wasn't. The little everyday worries that before had taken up a lot of my time became less and less important, and I found I became a much calmer person. It was difficult to explain what was happening or why, but a few months later I realised I had changed, and this time it had been so gradual I hadn't really noticed. And this is the thing: I realised I had never really noticed anything at all about myself before, about my shoulders, my walking, my breathing. I had been too busy going over and over what I had done or said, worrying what people were thinking about me. They were probably not interested, because they were also thinking about themselves. I slowly realised I had wasted my time doing this every day.

I continued my lessons, and read even more books and everything felt so different. I found my voice and said what I wanted to say. I no longer worried that it was not perhaps the right thing to say. I expressed my own opinions, and I felt more honest and happier for saying what I knew was right for me, even if it went against what someone else thought. I also realised that even though I had grown-up children, I had still felt like a child myself, not the real parent but just someone playing the part. Then I noticed as I was speaking to my daughter or son, or if I was on the phone at work, the voice I heard didn't sound like mine any more, but someone else's, sounded mature and confident, who knew exactly what they were saying. I noticed physical changes too. My feet were straighter when I walked – I had previously walked with my feet turned out in a ten-to-two position, and I began to become aware of a new sensation in my neck and shoulders. I also felt it was time to give up a habit I'd had for over thirty years of sitting on a cushion when I was driving. I had convinced myself that I couldn't drive without it. I took a chance, and I was quite safe!

Over the following months, and due to an increased awareness of everything around me, I came to believe that this was my particular way forward. It just felt right. Nothing else had grabbed my attention the way Alexander lessons had. The lessons were a haven. There was no negativity, no criticism, no need to worry if I was right or wrong, and this was something I had not experienced before.

Training to be an Alexander Technique teacher was the next change in direction for me. It was not a simple decision, with many personal and financial problems to overcome during the three years of training. But I proved to myself that if you remove the obstacles you place in your own way, anything is possible. I still have many days when I seem to be going backwards: the difference now is that I can let those thoughts go and move on. By coming back to what I can hear and what I can see, by feeling the ground under my feet, I am smiling again and feel so lucky to have discovered a fantastic way of living.

## Getting the Horse to Move
### Anonymous

I am a forty-seven-year-old hospital consultant and am a keen horsewoman, having my own horses. In 2010 I had had symptoms of pain, numbness and tingling down my left leg for just over two years. Initially a slipped disc was diagnosed, for which I had physiotherapy for about five or six months, to little effect. I also had a few sessions of Chinese acupuncture for the pain, but didn't feel it made any difference.

I subsequently became unable to stand up straight (though I felt that I was!). A repeat MRI scan showed that I now had a spondylolisthesis (where one vertebra slips forward relative to the one below it). An orthopaedic colleague offered facet joint injections for the pain (which I declined on the basis that I needed the pain to stop me doing things I shouldn't do that may further stress my back) and also said that it looked like I would need surgery to fuse part of my spine. This really worried me as it would mean losing part of my body's shock absorption mechanism. I had a few sessions of osteopathy but was less than impressed about its effectiveness for me.

At this point I was getting desperate! I knew about the Alexander Technique thanks to the eight-five-year-old teacher I go to with the horses, who has great posture having used the Alexander Technique for years.

The Alexander Technique 'fixed' me! Or should I say taught me how to direct and consciously use my body better. After about six lessons my back just got straighter and straighter, and the lump from the spondylolisthesis disappeared. I started thinking that maybe I just imagined that there had been a lump there at all, but there certainly isn't anymore! The pain, numbness and tingling had also gone – by lesson five.

I get an ache sometimes, particularly if I lie flat on something that has got no cushioning, but it usually wears off quite quickly because

I use what I have learnt in my AT lessons – Alexander Technique lengthening.

I ride using the principles of natural horsemanship (which I also teach) and classical riding. With both my aim is to work in harmony with the horse, endeavouring to help the horse use its body well and efficiently, from back to front, rather than forcing it (by pulling on the reins) to adopt a shape from the front end.

For my riding, the Alexander Technique has helped to make me much more consciously aware of what I'm doing, and how this influences what the horse does and how the horse is using its body. Whether I'm riding or working on the ground with the horses, if I'm tipping forward and sticking my pelvis out, they will drag their bum as well. Whereas, if I bring mine in, they'll engage and use themselves differently, such that if I'm working them at liberty, loose in the school and I'm on the ground, I can stop them just by releasing my lower back to tip my bum in, and they'll stop.

I am using my way of going to affect the horse's way of going. I always have done this to some degree, but by having that consciousness of being able to adjust and let go of tensions by thinking rather than doing something, it just seems to happen (mostly!!), and then you become aware that something in the horse has changed too, which is completely beyond my scientific training, but, it happens and is truly amazing. If things change for the better then it's cool.

I wish I had learnt Alexander Technique years ago! But hey, you shouldn't beat yourself up about what you didn't know. However you should beat yourself up if you know about something good/better but ignore it and continue doing what you've always done! I think AT lessons should be recommended to ALL riders.

## Twisting to the Right While Leaning to the Left
Richard Brennan

I first came to the Technique because of a back problem which was primarily caused by many years of work as a driving instructor. The sedentary position that I had adopted for up to ten hours a day did nothing for my posture, which became so hunched that I remember someone saying I looked like a person who had been living in a very small cottage with very low ceilings for a very long time! I often spent fifty hours a week sitting in a car with terrible seats, and it is not really surprising to me now that after several years I developed lower-back pain. At first it was an occasional aching back that was relieved by massage or some gentle exercise, but it got worse and worse; eventually I was suffering with an extremely painful condition. Often I could hardly walk with the pain. Although I did not know it, my quest to try and get relief for my painful and debilitating condition would take me on an incredible journey of self-discovery and change my direction in life.

Many people who have back problems make an appointment with their doctor and perhaps only spend a few minutes being examined, after which they are given painkillers, muscle relaxants or anti-inflammatories, or advised to rest. I know many people think that if the doctor had more time to examine them properly the treatment would be more effective. In my case, my father was a doctor and it was not a matter of a few minutes' examination – I had all the time I needed, but got the same treatment and advice (painkillers and I was told to rest). This, however, only brought temporary relief and, as time went by, even the powerful painkilling drugs I was taking became less and less effective. I remember him saying, 'If you ever want a day off work, just say you have back pain, because nobody can tell if you have, and nobody can tell if you haven't; and if you have, nobody can do anything about it!'

It was not long before I needed to get back to work due to financial pressures, but sitting in the car only made the problem worse, so I attended numerous physiotherapists. Although some of the treatments helped for a day or two, my condition got steadily worse. Before long I was also suffering with sciatic pains shooting down my left leg. I got to a stage where I could not sit, stand or walk without pain shooting through my whole body.

I saw a series of orthopaedic surgeons (some of the best in the country) who took X-rays and performed various other tests. Although a prolapsed disc was diagnosed as the cause of my problem, no one could tell me what had caused the disc to move out of position in the first place, or how I could get it back in place! I was merely told that I would have to get used to the fact that I would never be able to bend, lift or carry anything ever again. The surgeon advised me to undergo surgery to remove the three lowest intervertebral discs. This, he promised, would reduce the level of pain. I initially agreed to this, but my father persuaded me to cancel the operation because he was seeing people who had undergone similar operations, many of whom were in even more pain than before. Very few were actually any better. Fortunately, surgeons rarely perform this operation anymore because of its failure rate. So, looking back, I had a lucky escape.

The only other course of treatment left open to me was an intensive course of physiotherapy and, although it had not worked before, I went as a last desperate attempt to find some relief from the pain. I signed in as an inpatient at a large residential physiotherapy hospital near London, UK. One of the treatments at the hospital involved improving posture, and I was told to 'hold myself straight' and 'pull my shoulders back', but this only aggravated my pain instantly. In fact, it aggravated the problems of all the other patients in the session too. Although the physiotherapists and doctors were very concerned and obviously doing their best to help, the treatment and exercises they gave were not helping me at all (and by talking to other patients there, not many others either); in fact when I was discharged from the hospital my back pain was worse than ever.

At this stage I started to investigate various forms of alternative medicine. These included more established therapies such as chiropractic, osteopathy, homoeopathy and acupuncture. I then tried less orthodox treatments such as reflexology, yoga, metamorphic technique, aromatherapy, reiki, rebirthing and spiritual healing. In fact, at this point I was so desperate I would have tried practically anything. Some of these treatments were better than others, but I could get only short-term relief. The severe pain always returned within days of any treatment. I finally gave up after many years of searching and resigned myself to a life of pain. Up to this point no one, including myself, had questioned why the discs had become prolapsed in the first place. I was forced to give up work even though I had a young family to support – things were becoming more and more desperate.

One day, quite by chance, I met an Alexander Technique teacher who explained how the Alexander Technique could be effective in helping back sufferers like myself who had tried many other remedies without success. He talked to me for over an hour explaining what the Technique was, yet in the end I could not understand what on earth he was talking about! Although I still had no idea what it was, and was understandably very sceptical after all the other treatments I had received, I decided to have a couple of sessions to see what it was about. At this point I was still desperate. The pain was present day and night. I felt that I had nothing to lose. Before meeting this teacher I had come across the Technique in the context of music and acting. Being neither a musician nor an actor, I was not sure how it was going to help me.

Within minutes of starting my first lesson, he asked me, 'Do you always sit like that?' I replied, 'Sit like what?' I really did not understand what he was talking about until he placed a mirror in front of me and I could clearly see that I was twisting to the right while leaning at least twenty degrees to the left. Yet, despite the fact that I could clearly see that I was sitting in a very crooked way, I still 'felt' perfectly straight. This was quite a revelation to me. I was amazed that I had never noticed it before.

The teacher started to make a few gentle adjustments to the way I was sitting and two things happened: in my new position I felt completely twisted to the left while leaning way off to the right, yet at the same time my back pain started to ease. He showed me how I was sitting in the mirror and to my amazement I saw I was sitting perfectly straight.

## Unreliable Sensory Appreciation

After a few lessons the changes felt less strange when I was straight, and my back pain started, slowly but surely, to decrease. It was at this point I realised that when I had been teaching people to drive, I had developed the habit of leaning to the left while twisting my pelvis to the right, so that I could see both the road ahead and check to make sure that the learner driver was looking in his mirrors at the same time. Over time this had become my habit whenever I sat and it was this very tendency that had given me all my problems. As the tensions released during a series of lessons I also noticed that it was not only my back that was improving; I started to sleep better, my self-esteem and confidence also grew and, to my surprise, I was gradually becoming happier as well. Within twelve weeks of starting lessons I was leading a normal life again, lifting and bending without any problem at all.

I was so impressed with my recovery, especially as I had been 'written off' by so many other methods, that I went on a three-year course and trained to be an Alexander teacher myself. Today, thirty years later, I can honestly say that I have hardly had any back pain at all, and I am happy that I have been able to help many other people like me who have had back pain or other musculoskeletal conditions where no other treatment or technique has been able to make any difference. It is very satisfying, and a real privilege to help these people in the same way that I myself was helped.

There have been many other benefits that I personally have derived from the Alexander Technique, apart from the absence of back pain. I feel it has made me calmer and more appreciative of all that life has to offer, and able to cope with all the ups and downs that are a part of human existence. I was diagnosed with other health problems: within the space of four months I was found to have high blood pressure, high cholesterol levels, and type two diabetes. I then suffered a stroke.

I believe my training in the Alexander Technique helped me see that it was again unconscious habitual behaviour that had caused these problems. I decided very quickly that I did not want to carry a bag full of pills around with me for the rest of my life, and was determined that I was going to find the root cause of these problems.

With the help of a fascinating book called *The China Study*, I came to the conclusion that it was dietary habits that had caused my health problems. Overnight, I decided to completely change what I ate. I believe that that by changing my diet alone I was able to avoid further strokes, completely reverse the diabetes and reduce my cholesterol levels to below average. Not only that, but the daily Alexander sessions straight after my stroke greatly helped me get back to good health. I was working full time again in a matter of weeks.

*Unreliable Sensory Appreciation*

# Small Surprises When You Don't Expect Them
## Anne Landa

The Alexander Technique has been present in my life since I had a serious problem with my wrist. As an accordion player, when I was seventeen years old I developed tendonitis of my left wrist. Among other therapies, and after asking for a solution 'everywhere', a physiotherapist tried to help me by treating the inflammation with cortisone, so I could continue playing. Time passed, and my playing depended on how my wrist responded each time, for each repertoire and each different stimulus, connected to an unknown response. My wrist has been very vulnerable and my worry was always about it. I continued asking for information. In the meantime, a physiotherapist told me that my tendonitis had become chronic.

Some years later, I lived in Rome, where I played concerts, but my wrist was still hurting. For a musician having such a constant negative isn't comfortable. One day I found an Alexander Technique advertisement and I decided to try it, while being very sceptical.

From the beginning of my AT work with my first teacher, I realised that the problem wasn't my wrist! It was what I was doing with myself! AT lessons showed me clearly that I wanted to be involved in Alexander training.

I trained in Amsterdam between 1997 and 2001. After, I returned to Spain where my teaching started privately. Later, I initiated a teaching programme for AT in a conservatory (Musikene, Basque Country) in parallel with teaching AT and the accordion privately, in order to develop AT work for musicians in my country. I still give Alexander Technique lessons there, along with teaching the accordion.

But in October 2003, I suffered a terrible car accident (in a taxi, going to teach lessons in the music school). The taxi driver died and I suffered trauma to my head and face – broken socket of my right eye, a broken nose, broken upper jaw bones (both the right and left sides) – as well as a broken pelvic bone, and a broken ankle.

I slept in the intensive care unit for some days in an induced coma until it became possible to operate on my swollen face. Thanks to a tracheotomy, I could breathe through my trachea, and Dr Llop in Cruces Hospital in Bilbao was in charge of surgery that many specialists afterwards considered to be a great success. No doubt, in my opinion, the surgical aspect of the medicine has developed in such a way that human beings have to appreciate it.

My recovery has been a real journey, but I have to admit that from the moment I awoke in the hospital room after the operation, my body was so damaged that I realised that psychological power took over. Somehow I opened my eyes and saw who was there: I felt the happiest person in the world.

My conclusion is that when the physical side is so damaged, the psychological helps and gives you power to smile. Those moments were the happiest ones in my life, even if it sounds incredible.

The recovery was long, and at first the hardest was the tracheotomy and the problems associated with it when I couldn't breathe freely, nor could I talk. The feeling of having a 'hole' through which you breath, sometimes not freely because it is blocked by blood and other problems, causes huge interference in the whole system: the fear reflex is present and the shortening of the whole structure is immediate.

When the tracheotomy started to be less vulnerable, I felt stronger (even if I couldn't stand up). I remember one day I tried to stand when I found myself alone for a moment in my hospital bedroom. Mentally, I was sure I could stand up, but my proprioception didn't function properly, and I fell. I realised that I couldn't yet stand up. My mental orders were clear, but my body was not able and wasn't ready yet: I didn't have any support from my musculature. When many parts in our bodies are broken somehow the wholeness gets disconnected.

During my recovery after leaving the hospital, I had to lie down for some months to allow the broken bones of my pelvis to reattach themselves to their natural location. Not moving or standing was the only way to allow the bones to find their place again. In the meantime,

## Unreliable Sensory Appreciation

my ankle had been immobile for too long, causing a limitation in the range of movement. After long months practising, I learnt to walk again and while the physiotherapists were insistent about the position of my feet, I remember thinking, 'my head leading' in my little first steps. Many months exercising in tepid water was a good training as well, to develop my musculature and connect my parts into a 'whole'.

My eye socket and face bones were pinned in the right place with titanium plates, but the connection of the trigeminal nerve to my upper lip was damaged, which caused partial paralysis and a loss of feeling in the upper lip. Even today, this remains, and I have limited movement in my maxillary, temporal and frontal face bones because of mucus. Osteopathy helps.

The broken eye socket resulted in diplopia. But the diplopia, even though it remains today, was not such a problem after I realised that the best solution was to articulate the head from the atlanto-occipital joint and, going down the stairs (where I see double), just moving my head to avoid that angle.

The ophthalmologist told me once that the ease with which I could move my head in every direction was great(!); this was the result of just thinking of releasing my neck and my head going forward and up.

I remember, even in the hospital bed, that I was thinking about my neck being free, and somehow my system was alert to my thinking. I didn't decide to think about it at any point, it just came.

I visited a physiotherapist and osteopath: her opinion was that it is incredible that I don't have migraines, cervical problems and there are no problems with the sacrum at all. She thought that the medical team treating me had done a fantastic job. Then I told her that I'm an Alexander Technique teacher, and it is clear to me that my sensitivity to proprioception helped me a lot in my journey, a journey that hasn't finished, of course. During the autumn of 2013, I had another operation to take a piece of titanium and five screws from my facial bones (twenty-five screws still remain in place...) that were causing problems with my teeth. It was hard to go back to my surgeon, and to consciously choose to enter the operating theatre. But it was, shall we say, the 'last chapter'.

I would like to say a special thanks to my AT training teachers, and to my first Alexander teacher. Thanks to whole my family and my love, of course! And to the important persons in my life.

For the first time after seven years, I drove a car. I drove my baby to her music lesson. It took me a long time to get to the point where, realising that the fear was there, suddenly I felt I could drive again.

Dr. Chouza, my psychiatrist, helped me to free my mind to try and control the fear. I was convinced that I would never drive again. Today, I know that I am able to drive, but I have to use my consciousness to control, not my own fear of driving, but the worry of being hurt by another driver. For that reason, I prefer to drive only when necessary.

Our mental state is the most important element, no doubt about it.

Almost twelve years have passed. I am the mother of a girl and a boy, and am pregnant again (the baby due in the autumn of 2015). I never would have imagined having three babies; it was a very clear decision for me, because now I know that life happens just once, and you've got to go for whatever you feel is important – we don't know where we're going to be tomorrow.

My first baby (2008) was delivered in hospital because I was afraid, due to my broken pelvis. Even if everything seemed to be fine, I didn't dare have her at home. My second baby (2012) was delivered at home, and even though he was in a posterior position, by crawling I delivered him quite easily, and the dilatation went perfectly in 'monkey'. So, since 2003, the unity of my primary control has given me more power in all senses of the word.

I think now that the Alexander Technique development of oneself is full of small surprises which come when you don't expect them, and our 'leitmotiv' is the key: STOP and THINK.

Slowly the episode of the accident has given me the consciousness to be in the present, and slowly I want to bring to the fore of my memory the hours that I have forgotten, and that are not part of myself. Nowadays I try (without end-gaining) to remember what happened before and after the accident; slowly images come. Don't fear: stop and think, and it will come, because it is part of my life and my mind has it hidden somewhere...

I realised that our mind is our treasure: our conscious control comes from there. So, the more we stop, the more we react as we really are. And after a traumatic experience, our mind needs time, space and trust to be open again: somehow I experienced a 'closing door' in my mind (fear of the environment). Now, thanks to my babies as well as the experience of delivery at home, thanks to love around me and music, this 'door' in my mind is opening slowly, as if saying, 'welcome to the world again'.

# Working Through the Contractions
## Katie Dixon

I am a clinical psychologist and mother of two sons.

Long before their births, I'd been having this problem of stiffness and aching in my neck. There was a lot going on at the time for me. I'd had a miscarriage, and I was just at a point where I was thinking, 'I need to have a look at the way that I'm living my life' and 'Do I need to look after myself a bit better?' It occurred to me that I could actually go and have something done about this neck problem. I'd just been living with it, really. I was talking about it to my brother, who'd had lessons, and he said 'Why don't you try the Alexander Technique?' He bought me my first lesson as a birthday present.

I certainly think there were benefits, in both the physical and mental areas. I feel much more aware. I was already aware that stress and tension played a large part in the neck problem, but it made me even more aware of the micro-level of tension. I could do usual sort of relaxation stuff, but as I learned the Alexander Technique I became aware of this almost-unnoticeable tightening while I was doing things. There was a broader benefit as well. I felt I was looking after myself a bit more.

It helped that I could use the Technique when I got pregnant. Unfortunately, it helped me less the first time I gave birth than the second time, even though I was actually having lessons during the first pregnancy. The first delivery was induced because my waters broke, and there were no contractions. There was meconium in the waters, which can be a sign of foetal distress, so I was stuck in the bed and couldn't really get into the positions I wanted. In that respect, I was disappointed that I hadn't been able to use the Technique a bit more, really. In the earlier stages, I was able to use it, and I had to, as the induced contractions were horrendously painful. As it happened, the baby was fine.

In my second delivery, I had the same thing (the waters going and no contractions) but that time there wasn't any meconium, so they were happy to see what happened over the next twenty-four hours. The birth happened naturally after a few hours anyway. I was more able to move around and keep upright. There is something about lying down: it's strange, because it is so often seen as being the position that you are supposed to give birth in, but there was something about being in the upright position that meant that I could concentrate a bit more, particularly on my neck and shoulders and keep them loose, and also concentrate on my breathing a bit more. I felt I was able to work through the contractions better, whereas the first time I was just kind of surviving and enduring them.

# The Tree Branch
Anonymous

One day, when I was five or six years old, I was told by my mum not to go out, but my sister decided that we would go out and play on a tree which had a swing hanging from a horizontal branch. My sister had the idea, so she was first up on the branch and she had the baby on her arm. I had to get up there as well, but I had to use the swing to climb up. I couldn't do it, so she was holding the baby with one hand and was trying to pull me up. I fell. I broke my left upper arm and dislocated the shoulder. For three days I was in pain but I didn't dare tell. One day, I had to put my hands up in the air for Mum to get my dress on, and I couldn't do it. Then she knew something was wrong, and in anger ripped the dress from the shoulder down and there it was, black and blue.

In 1972, in London, I was working in the fur trade, making heavy mink coats. One coat had about a thousand mink in it. When I had hung it up, I couldn't move, my left arm was stuck. So the forelady had to come and move me. I was taken to the fracture clinic in London, and they said they 'didn't know what had happened but it was the result of a childhood injury'. I was put in a collar and given traction and heat treatment to the neck. There was awful pain down the arm into the hand. I didn't sleep for seven nights, though I was on DF118 (a very strong painkiller). Even that worked only for two hours; I was in continuous pain. I am black, but my skin was whiter than the sheets because I could not sleep and because of the pain. I could move my arm but the pain was really, really bad. There was not much more they could do for me. I got hands-on therapy and did all sorts of exercises with a stick and things like that, and eventually it did get easier. It took quite some time to get back to normal. They said I had to give up the machining because holding my neck bent forwards all the time wasn't doing the neck or the arm any good.

They would have written me off as medically unfit but I couldn't face that, so I gave up the machining, and went to work in a hospital. I moved to Leicester and everything was fine. Then suddenly it was changed from a hospital to an old people's home.

One day in 1992, another carer and I put somebody into a chair, and when I went to turn back, I was standing but I could not feel my legs whatsoever and had pain in my lower back. So, off I went to the infirmary, and the doctor said that the problem was in my neck. There was pain down the left arm again. So I had all sorts of treatment and it got better again.

From then on my back got really and truly bad. Sometimes I was standing and, apart from pain, I couldn't feel my legs. So they sent me for an MRI which showed spondylolisthesis at the fourth and fifth lumbar vertebrae. They decided to retire me, and I decided to relocate to Barbados in 2002. One night in 2003 I woke up with excruciating pain inside the left shoulder blade, and I realised that my left arm was completely paralysed. I couldn't move it, I couldn't raise it. I had lots of pain. The fingers were floppy, there was no feeling in them, and the palm was hooked. Within about three weeks, my fourth and fifth fingers improved but the first two fingers and thumb were still not right. In about 2009, I fell down, broke the ring finger and dislocated the little finger. The front was twisted toward the back. The pain was so bad that when I saw it, I just grabbed it and spun it around back into place. It was four months before I actually got to have another MRI, and was diagnosed with a brachial plexus lesion.

I had the same paralysis until this year. When I went to see the physiotherapist, they gave me no hands-on work, just a paper with hand exercises and no follow-up. So I asked my doctor to refer me to an occupational therapist. He said to me 'go to Boots and explain' and they would sell me a splint.

I kept visiting the GP and was eventually referred to an occupational therapist. She made up a sort of splint to match the shape of the hand and to help straighten it out. Well, she did as much as she could, but it didn't do a lot. She gave me a bottle to pump with the hand. At first, I couldn't do it, but eventually I could. I went to stay with my daughter because at that time I couldn't dress or do anything for myself. I bought a wax machine and a TENS machine. I bought a hand grip exerciser, but I couldn't use it. Then I started going to a Chinese acupuncturist. I had cupping; I had massage. These things helped a little with the pain but not with the movement. This went on for eighteen months. The acupuncturist said I would have to have a break, so after nine months' break, I went again. I began to think it was a waste of money, and I started doing lots of things myself with it. I even made a sling and used to make it pull the arm up and down. I used to do all sorts of things to try to improve matters.

I worked in the hospital's geriatric department and I was familiar with rehabilitation, because I had to take patients down there from the ward. I did all the rehabilitation things I saw being done on my patients, and I worked on the hand myself. Before I had Alexander Technique lessons, I went to an osteopath, but unfortunately, although she helped me with my back there was nothing she could do with the hand. Well, I told her not to worry about the left hand as it seemed hopeless, but I needed help as I was getting a lot of pain in the right hand. She said to me the right hand was overworked and there is nothing more she could do for me. I went and had more cupping and acupuncture and then went back again to see the osteopath about a year later, and she said to me, 'I'm sorry, there is nothing I can do for you, but if you are willing, I will send you to somebody who will sort you, because the whole of your back is out of line', so that's when she recommended a teacher for Alexander Technique lessons.

I looked in the mirror and saw the bodily misalignment for myself. Although I had only nine lessons in three months, I could see that my head was straighter. I could see the difference in the mirror. I still have the pain in my left arm, but the pain in the right hand is much less. Before the lessons, the fingers of my left hand were deformed. They were all bent and wouldn't straighten. After three lessons they were straight. The index finger is not one hundred percent, but the thumb and the little finger are. The sensation is a lot easier in the fingers, but not in the shoulder. The little finger and ring finger are still numb. I am used to that (that happened when I broke the fingers), but I have got some feeling back already.

*Unreliable Sensory Appreciation*

The usage of the whole left arm has changed. I am able to do things. I could not grip with my left hand. Since I have had the lessons, I can lift my hand and I can comb my hair, where I could not comb my hair at all because the left hand would not reach up. At mealtimes I was cutting everything up with my right hand and then taking a fork to eat with my right hand. Now I am eating with a knife and fork. If I wanted to wash my tights, I used only the right hand, but now the left hand can do everything that the right hand can, not as well or as strong, but it is cooperating: the two hands work together. Before I had lessons, I couldn't peel potatoes because my left hand couldn't hold the potato peeler or potato. So I didn't peel potatoes, I washed them. But now, I choose whether I want potatoes in their jacket or I can peel them. I chop up beans and do a lot of things that I couldn't do before.

The Technique has made a lot of difference psychologically. I was frustrated most of the time, going to the hairdressers to have my hair done because I could not style it or put it up. Now I can. It helped me to be able to dress myself: I couldn't tie my laces, pull a zip with my left hand, or manage buttons. So it has helped me to do things in general, and I feel better about myself, about how I look and how I care about myself.

# Discovering the Liberated Breath
Simon Spire

The first time I remember becoming conscious of my breathing mechanism was when I was about nine years old. As my family sat around the dinner table in Auckland, New Zealand, my father – who was often stressed and regularly searching for ways to counter his stress – shared that he had just learned from a breathing expert that we should ideally take only eight full breaths per minute. I tested myself and noticed that I had difficulty achieving this. Clearly, I thought, it was something I would have to work on.

My passing attempt to implement it now seems to presage the long line of misguided battles I would later wage on my breath as an adult, a struggle that would revolve around the symptoms of 'air hunger' and chronic chest-breathing, and that would be complicated by the imperfect tool known as 'belly-breathing.'

I was for the most part happily oblivious to the rhythm of my breath until I reached the age of seventeen. It was then that I began to notice a sensation of being starved for breath, something that I would come to know as 'air hunger.' It was only mild, and so it didn't cause too much of a distraction; whenever I noticed that I was starved for air, my immediate reaction would be to take a big breath in my chest. It felt almost as if I were forcing myself to yawn in order to satisfy this urge for more air.

The phenomenon became more pronounced, however, over the following two years. In hindsight, I'm sure that the onset of this breathing pattern was the consequence of my increasingly imbalanced approach to life. I had become almost wholly focused on the future, driven both by ambition and fear to doggedly pursue some ideal of success. It had become normal for me to exist in a highly accelerated and hyper-analytical mode. Still, this was only the tip of the iceberg: on a more primary level I felt lost, empty and stifled, and was struggling to make sense of life.

## Unreliable Sensory Appreciation

I searched relentlessly for something to fill the void, a dynamic that was apparently mirrored on a physical level in my frantic and frustrating efforts to satisfy my body's craving for air. I believe that other factors – such as weight-training, breathing exercises for singing and vague instructions I had received on 'diaphragmatic breathing' – also contributed to the onset of these breathing difficulties, albeit to a lesser degree.

At the age of eighteen, the growing discomfort surrounding my breathing had reached a point where it was a constant presence in my life. I had developed a chronic habit of trying to satisfy the urge for air by reaching for a breath in a forced and unnatural way. However, the muscle tension involved in this strained breathing ultimately exacerbated the sense of being starved for air. This created a self-reinforcing pattern that would leave me feeling even more uncomfortable than before. At that point I would have to tolerate the feelings of air hunger for a number of hours before my reaching for air would once again be effective. But even when it was effective, it provided only momentary relief; the sensation of being starved for air persisted regardless of what I did. I developed significant tension in my chest, neck, shoulders and jaw, and the feelings of discomfort and struggle that accompanied this breathing complication were abiding. I would occasionally be unaware of the tension when distracted by an activity or conversation, but only sometimes, and it would never last. Although the subjective experience was one of constant struggle and primal discomfort, the extent of the problem was not particularly discernible from the outside in any dramatic way and everyday life continued normally.

Early on, I sought help from a breathing specialist with a background in physiotherapy who made a number of helpful observations: I was relying too heavily on my chest for my breathing; the position of my chin was too high; and the muscles of my upper back, neck, chest and shoulders carried considerable tension. I learned about my habit of 'chest-breathing,' its inefficiency and the function of the diaphragm in natural breathing. I learned that I was not exhaling fully, and was instead inhaling new air on top of stale air. She diagnosed my condition as 'hyperventilation syndrome' and named the symptoms 'air hunger.'

The solution that I was given to address my faulty breathing was the technique of belly-breathing, sometimes called diaphragmatic breathing. I was taught to focus the movement of my breath in the abdominal area. I was also told that my chest shouldn't move during effective breathing. Attention was also given to my exhalations and my abdomen was encouraged to contract as part of that to ensure that I was exhaling fully. The last significant components of the prescription were to 'tuck' my tailbone forward and allow my shoulders to relax forward, rather than trying to hold them back.

As my symptoms worsened, my breathing battle intensified. On the one hand, I was diligently practicing belly-breathing and ensuring that my chest did not move, while on the other hand, I had developed a strong habit of chest-breathing that desperately wanted to be satisfied. The belly-breathing I had been taught never seemed to provide a satisfying breath, and overriding the habit of chest-breathing was an awful task, because it felt like I was truly starving myself of air. It was clear that I was definitely not in alignment with my natural breathing mechanism. Still, believing that I was getting the best advice possible, I continued to practice what I was taught, and was told that it just required repetition and a gradual phasing-out of my habit of chest-breathing.

At the age of nineteen, after two years of worsening symptoms since first encountering air hunger, I saw my GP to ask if he could shine any light on the situation. I relayed what I had been taught. He seemed somewhat hesitant about my assertion that the chest should not move during correct breathing and referred me to an ENT specialist, who decided that perhaps surgery on my sinuses and turbinates could assist with my breathing, given that I had a history of mild allergies. As much as it makes me wince today, I went ahead and had surgery in the hope that I would find relief from my breathing difficulties. The surgery appeared to reduce my mild allergy symptoms, but failed to have any impact on my breathing problems.

The worst of my symptoms continued until, at the age of twenty-one, I found a second breathing specialist in my hometown of Auckland who finally offered a piece of advice that provided the beginning of real relief. She suggested that my problems were probably the result of stress and anxiety causing my sympathetic nervous system to be overactive, which eventually led to chest-breathing becoming an engrained habit. It was the simplest and most accurate explanation I had heard. I had been hopeful that the symptoms of air hunger would subside as my emotional state improved, but this hadn't been the case, and I wanted to understand what more I could do.

This new specialist told me that the physical habits would stay in place until they were broken, despite my having moved through the personal struggles that may have caused the habits in the first place. She offered me the one piece of advice that finally, after four years, began to free me of the habit of chest-breathing, of gasping for air and of the perpetual sensation of needing to force a tense and panicked yawn to inhale enough air. She made it clear that the only solution was to completely override the habit of satisfying that need for air, to refuse to give in to the habit to any degree or in any way.

It took all of my willpower to consistently override my body's impulse to get the air it sought through reaching. As much as I hated the feelings of struggling for air that had plagued me for years, this was even worse: now I felt starved of air – which was nothing new – but I also had to suppress my body's desire to grasp for that air. Sometimes it felt like I was literally suffocating myself by not following the impulse to take a chest breath, and what was more, I had to be vigilant about it at all times; I could never allow myself a 'rest'. Whenever I did allow myself this relief, I would notice that the habit would once again gather momentum and I would be back at square one. The specialist was right: I couldn't cut corners if I wanted to be free of these problems.

Eventually, discovering a new sense of resolve, I managed a full month without once giving in to the impulse to reach for air. The impulse to reach for air was still alive in me, but it was no longer in control. My breathing did not feel comfortable, but I was at last no longer helplessly attempting to satisfy my craving for air. It was as if a debilitating addiction had been overcome, and it was a huge relief to finally be free of it. I was overjoyed to realise that I had freed myself from a burden that I had begun to believe would be with me for the rest of my life.

For several years my breathing remained relatively stable yet persistently uncomfortable. While I had overcome the chronic chest-breathing and reaching for breath that I had come to know as the worst of my symptoms, the sense of air hunger remained. So, too, did the impulse to force myself to yawn, though it was no longer controlling me. My dysfunctional breathing was now more tolerable, though the core problems persisted: my breathing felt stifled, restricted and unnatural, and it seemed that something that was for most people unconscious and effortless was still problematic and a frequent distraction for me.

Over the years, I searched for a solution to my breathing difficulties, at times in tandem with my search for answers regarding my voice. As a singer, I would often strain or lose my voice. I received acupuncture, saw a chiropractor, tried massage and consulted various natural health practitioners. Having by this stage moved to California and later New York, there was no shortage of options. I also explored a number of different exercise modalities, many of which ended up actually exacerbating the tension I experienced in my breathing. Nothing worked. No matter what I did, the discomfort and air hunger remained.

I had encountered the Alexander Technique in my research, and decided to see if it could assist with my breathing and postural confusion. I found a nearby teacher whom I would later discover had a special interest in the breathing mechanism, and it didn't take long for me to know that I was finally on the right track.

Over the course of my first few lessons, I became impressed with the wisdom and efficacy of the approach. Viewing the body as innately capable of balance and efficiency, the potential for imbalance and inefficiency was attributed to our own learned habits that ran counter to the body's natural intelligence. Or, as F. M. Alexander himself put it, 'The right thing does itself.' This resonated with me. I needed to identify the habits I had built that had come to interfere with the body's natural breathing mechanism, and then free myself from those habits.

Furthermore, instead of isolating a particular part of a system, or focusing on the symptom instead of the cause, the Alexander Technique considered the system as a whole. In my case, for example, breathing was not dealt with in isolation. It was understood in relation to what I was doing with the rest of my body, from my feet, to my hips, to my head and everywhere in between. Interfering with my body's natural movement in the way I held my head, for example, would have an impact on other parts of my body involved in breathing.

The fundamental difference between the Alexander Technique and everything that I had explored earlier was the perspective of 'inhibiting' my learned habits, and in doing so, allowing the body's natural efficiency to be restored. In contrast, my years of belly-breathing attempted to replace one habit (chest-breathing) with another, less harmful habit (belly-breathing). Although I found belly-breathing preferable to chest-breathing, I began to understand that it was still interfering with my body's natural breathing process. By identifying habits and then choosing not to reinforce them, the Alexander Technique enabled me to gradually rediscover my body's natural ease, free of the tension and inefficiency caused by my intervention. The undoing of habitual interference, combined with my teacher's guidance and direction, allowed the natural efficiency of my body to reawaken.

I was so excited by the truly holistic and logical approach of the Technique that I went for frequent lessons during my first three months. Each lesson, I would become more aware of my deeply entrenched habits and, with my teacher's guidance, I would experience the liberation of momentarily releasing those habits. It was the freest I could ever remember feeling in my body. So practised and deeply unconscious had my habits become, however, that they would invariably reassert themselves. I realised early on that there was always further to go; in peeling back one layer of habit, another more subtle layer was usually revealed before too long.

Perhaps even more important was recognising the tendency for new interfering habits to develop in response to the release of existing habits. I was continually surprised by how normal it was for me to attempt to 'do' the unlearning of my habits, responding to a genuine release of interference by then attempting to replicate it through remembering how I thought I 'did' it. The irony was, of course, that it was my doing that was the problem in the first place. In order to allow the natural intelligence to re-establish itself, I had to give up my attempts to interfere, even when the interference was well-intentioned. I found this particular parallel to certain Eastern philosophies of non-doing, surrender and non-resistance fascinating. The Alexander Technique, it seemed to me, could be viewed as an experiential parallel to these concepts, wherein the body's free use was a microcosm of and a metaphor for free awareness.

My breathing began to change. I started to experience greater ease in my body and in my breathing. As my habitual patterns gradually subsided, I began to discover the relief and freedom of a natural breath – something that perhaps I hadn't experienced since I was a young child. The initial discoveries afforded me by the Alexander Technique led more deeply into work that was specifically breath-focused. Work with Jessica Wolf's *The Art of Breathing*, which draws on both the Alexander Technique and the work of Carl Stough, was the most powerful tool I encountered for unlocking my body's natural, free breath. As my study continued, my breathing began moving toward a place of greater effortlessness and satisfaction.

The habitual compression of my chest – the result of years of following belly-breathing instructions that taught that my chest should not move and that I should encourage my abdomen to contract for the exhalation – eventually eased. However, whereas this chest-opening would have previously been impossible without triggering my forced-yawn and 'reaching' impulses, now this tension could be released without my body reverting back to this old habit, the Alexander principles of inhibition and direction providing the means for this. I was amazed by the freedom of breath that naturally emerged. It was true that there was a generous amount of movement in my abdomen, but now this was happening automatically and with greater freedom. Instead of this happening with the assistance of my abdominal muscles, which I realised I had been unknowingly engaging in my efforts to belly-breathe, it was now being freely propelled by the movement of my diaphragm. The same was true of my lower ribs, which began to gently swing as the lower lungs expanded, rather than being pulled open forcibly as in my previous habit of engaging the intercostals.

My diaphragm, being an involuntary muscle, was gradually redeveloping its natural resilience as we removed the impediments to its movement, namely my extraneous muscular tension. This recognition that the diaphragm was an involuntary muscle, and that it could not be controlled directly, was an important distinction. Whereas my earlier instruction in belly-breathing claimed to be engaging and utilising my diaphragm more fully, what I realised it had really been doing was encouraging my abdominal muscles to do some of the work that was naturally of the diaphragm's domain, creating greater interference in my natural breathing process.

As the strength of my habits diminished and I learned to trust the natural breath, I would occasionally experience tremors in my abdomen and chest. I came to understand this as a process of reclaiming areas of the natural range of movement that had been dormant for many years. These moments of liberation involved a natural expansion of my torso that took me beyond the territory I had previously known, providing a deeply satisfying, full breath, but without the tension of the need to 'grab' the air. I had to be careful not to interfere with this movement, as any muscular involvement on my part would cause unnecessary tension which would then restrict the full potential of the movement. Breath this satisfying depended on my being vigilant enough to give up the habitual impulses to 'do something' with my breathing.

My whole torso began to change. My back became fuller (in Alexander terminology, it lengthened and widened), providing support for the three-dimensional expansion of my torso that accompanied each inhalation, and for the corresponding movement of the exhalation. One day, after being seated for some time in a naturally poised position while meditating, I noticed my breath naturally seeking greater expansion in my upper back and chest. As I allowed the breath to guide my movement, my upper back, chest and shoulders seemed to naturally expand (widen) and move to what might be considered a more traditionally 'correct' postural position. It now felt as though my shoulders were further back than they had been for many years, though there was no muscular tension involved. Now, it seemed, the release of my habits had provided the space for my body to realign itself, and this extra capacity in my torso was being realised by my body as the breath naturally expanded into its full potential. The corresponding change in my breathing was, again, truly liberating and exhilarating.

One final realisation that has been particularly beneficial is understanding just how subdued the natural breath can be during times of minimal activity. I noticed how strong my tendency was to think that deep movement needs to be happening in order for the breath to be full. What I found, however, was that the free breath can often involve only very subtle – yet effortlessly coordinated – movement depending on the situation, and that allowing myself to be guided by this effortless rhythm rather than feeling that 'something had to be happening' actually resulted in some of the most potent moments of releasing habitual interference. I find it useful to remember that sometimes allowing the breath to be free means that there will be very little movement as entrenched restrictions are subtly unwound, and that permitting this process to unfold on its own schedule can be transformative.

After two or three years, satisfying breathing had become my norm. Remnants of tension still impeded my full breath at times, but this tension gradually subsided as the power of the underlying habits did. It was, and continues to be, an ongoing journey of discovering greater ease. My breathing became better than I had ever known it to be, and I am for the most part free of any distraction or discomfort stemming from breathing. Breathing has become enlivening, natural and enjoyable.

Looking back on the onset of my breathing difficulties at about age seventeen, I can see that my natural breathing pattern had become disrupted by the subconscious interference of my emotional state. My early habits were artificially exaggerating my body's natural breathing movements and creating real problems, and the well-intentioned instructions I was given early on were designed to combat these exaggerated movements. The conflict this created, however, ultimately compounded my difficulties. I believe that my experience demonstrates that substituting new habits for old habits is often not helpful and can be damaging. Rather, the habits must be addressed on a fundamental level and as part of the whole, while supporting the natural intelligence of the body to lead the way. For me, this was made possible by the Alexander Technique.

The Alexander Technique revealed that the secret to the battle with my breath was that there was no winning the war. In the conflict between my will and my habits, neither side could ever be victorious for long. However, what an exquisite surprise it was to discover that there need not be a winner in order for there to be peace. In exploring the opportunity to give up the struggle altogether, I discovered the resolve and understanding that enabled me to recognise my inadvertent perpetuation of this war, and then to gradually choose to surrender that. What was left in place of the conflict was the natural ease and intelligence of the body. My breath was finally liberated.

## Sending Directions

> *Supposing that the 'end' I decided to work for was to speak a certain sentence, I would start in the same way as before and (1) inhibit any immediate response to the stimulus to speak the sentence, (2) project in their sequence the directions for the primary control which I had reasoned out as being best for the purpose of bringing about the new and improved use of myself in speaking, and (3) continue to project these directions until I believed I was sufficiently au fait with them to employ them for the purpose of gaining my end and speaking the sentence. (The Use of the Self, 1932, p. 45)*

Sending directions is a mental activity of a particular kind which has an effect on the particular parts of the body involved in those directions. One example is Alexander's primary directions, 'Let the neck be free to let the head go forward and up to lengthen and widen the back', which, expressed slightly differently (and using the concept of inhibition) implies inhibiting the tendency to contract the neck and compress the spine. However, it can be much more than just physical. Directing our mind, body and life amounts to projecting something that is larger than us, stretching the envelope of life and changing our entire self and body image. Once we tap into what is beyond, we can tend in that direction without feeling that we must inevitably 'arrive' and without fear of failure.

Julia Buccetti says that she 'had always thought that my body carried me around, not that I carried my body around or that I could control it'. Lessons allowed her to realise 'how much easier stuff could be if

I lengthened myself and how much freer, how much stronger I could be'.

Melody Hirst treasures a particular memory: 'the first time I went on a long hill walk shortly after beginning the Alexander Technique, I followed my teacher's advice to remember "head, neck and back" as I walked and to be conscious of my body throughout the walk.'

Being present, being engaged – directing ourselves 'toward' – allows flexibility and grace, fluidity and adaptability in action and in life.

# Massage Therapy, Kick Boxing and Pole Dancing
## Julia Buccetti

I am a twenty-six-year-old massage therapist and pole-dance teacher, and I enjoy kick boxing, pole dancing and cycling as hobbies. I train a lot. I was doing kick boxing four times a week as well as pole dancing four times a week. I think I was even doing trampolining at the point when I started Alexander lessons, I was running, and I'm a massage therapist as well. And I cycle – everywhere.

The Alexander Technique teacher at the clinic where I work asked me if I would like to have some free lessons. I thought the lessons were absolutely amazing. I think I regained control of my body. I had always thought that my body carried me around, not that I carried my body around or that I could control it.

I got a lot out of my lessons. I realised how much easier stuff could be if I lengthened myself and how much freer, how much stronger I could be. I was able to allow the energy to pass through me instead of cutting it off. Training became much easier. I became more confident in my body and what it could do when I just relaxed about it and let it do its job. If I let it go, then I got so much more output than when I tried just to control power without actually letting power go through me. I found that I used the Alexander Technique before I would fight or compete, and that was really good. It relaxed my nerves.

It's been absolutely amazing in pole dancing because it has given me the ability to perform certain moves which I had written off as impossible because I was not flexible enough, like back bends, certain movements on the pole, a fish roll, even just doing the splits on the pole. Using the Alexander Technique and being able to do these movements, I have virtually opened up a whole new world for myself knowing that, 'Yes, I am capable of these moves because I have been able to improve my flexibility'. I have the confidence to say, 'Yes, you know what? My body can do these things', and it's really exciting.

I use it in cycling and that's been really good too. One thing that always stays with me is that the teacher told me to free my eyes; so now when I need to look up, I just lift my eyes and don't stiffen my neck to pull my head back. The Alexander Technique improved the speed and ease of cycling.

Everything I apply the Alexander Technique to is easier. In kick-boxing class we were doing 'floor to ceiling', where you touch the floor and then jump up to the touch the ceiling. We were told to do fifty. I have never been able to do fifty in one go; I would have to break and rest, and it was the first time ever that I was able to do fifty (which nobody else could do), and I did it using the Alexander Technique.

My teacher took me down to the park and showed me how to run when I was preparing for my first half marathon. Again, it just made my body lighter. I didn't seem to be carrying so much weight. Being able to have something to come back to or giving your directions kind of takes your mind away from the 'gruel' of it, and before you know it, you've been directing for twenty to forty minutes and you're like, 'Oh no way, I've done all this distance!', because it kind of takes you away. It makes time go; it makes running easier. You kind of go off somewhere. It's really, really good!

So there was my stretching as well. Now I really, really use it with my stretching. I would stretch after a session, I stretched for an hour the other day and it didn't feel like an hour at all but, because I was really taking my time and using the Alexander Technique, I could not believe it when I looked at the clock. Normally I would stretch for ten minutes, and at an hour I was like 'Wow'.

I did lie down in semi-supine before my pole-dance competitions. I found it a lot easier to use the Alexander Technique during a performance. Because I was not so rushed, I knew what I was doing and I could take my time, and I know where I was lengthening. I can practise that during the actual move. A fight isn't choreographed, so it seems much more rushed. I think that's my ultimate challenge, to be able to use Alexander within something that is so sporadic and panicky and rushed, because I think it will buy me that time, or get me into that time-free zone: that's really what I need to be able to do, take my time and pace it.

The physical benefit has been absolutely amazing and has given me confidence in my body. I felt like I was limited before; I don't feel limited physically at all now. Also, mentally it has given me so much more confidence, to be able to regain control, not just over my body, but also over my emotions. Because I know that, if I feel panicky, I can do the 'Whispered Ah'.

That also helped me not to restart smoking. It made me a lot calmer. I feel a lot calmer within my normal everyday life, emotionally, because I can combat stress in a much better way, and I have started using my lying down even more now. I feel that it is not just the physical aspect at all; my mental wellbeing, my emotional wellbeing. I used to have counselling. Since I started learning the Alexander Technique, I haven't felt the need. Though my counselling sessions are finished, I have felt quite content and know that, if I ever feel disturbance, I can always go back to the Alexander Technique, and it's something that I can do by myself, which is really, really nice.

The only bad thing I would say is that is has taken me so long (thirty lessons). I think I'm only starting to realise now that I am in control of the Alexander Technique. Whereas I did rely heavily on my teacher. I think she was a magician, in being able to allow my body to react and have these responses, and I associated that with having the lessons. But now I feel, 'No, it is something that I can do by myself and it works just as well'. It is empowering: I'm a magician too! It is very, very nice, but I still feel like I need the teacher, because the further I get with it the more questions I have. If I'd had five and stopped, I wouldn't have continued with it, but the more I've continued with lessons the more I've continued to use it, and the more I apply it to everything. I want to be able to apply it to literally everything that I do.

I know that it works, I know it does, because it does! If you apply it, if you use it. But you have to use it.

# 'No' is Not a Negative
## Rosemary Nott

In around 1948, when I was nineteen years old, I happened on one of F.M. Alexander's books in Chelsea Public Library – what an extraordinary chance, I often think now, not only that I idly pulled out that particular book, but that that particular book was there at all. I stood reading little passages here and there, thinking, 'Well, this makes sense'. It seemed like a little light was being thrown on what was becoming a rather dark horizon in my life. Some months earlier, I had stepped up to get on a train on my way to Art School, and not only stepped up, but seized up with excruciating pain in my lower back. Friends already in the carriage somehow hauled me in. This moment passed, and was quite quickly forgotten.

Then it happened again. And again. And memory and fear crept in. I began to have some vague idea of what 'positions' or 'postures' to take to avoid these painful episodes. A dull lower backache began to take up residence. Eventually, doctors, X-rays and physios took over. Exercises involving walking along a balance form (in retrospect, why?) gave me wicked cramps. Nothing that was tried, including electrical treatment in a footbath, 'worked'.

This was 1949 and few alternatives to the orthodox were widely known or available. Around this time I had met Adam Nott – eventually my husband to be – and his mother, both of whom had had lessons with F.M. not long before he died. Mrs Nott said she had heard that Alexander's niece, Marjory, and her doctor husband were starting up a practice near the Royal Albert Hall in London, and that they might be able to help my, by now miserable, back.

'Why not go and see them?' she said. So I made an appointment – little knowing that that phone call would change the whole direction of my life. In fact, halfway down the entrance stairs, I nearly turned tail – whatever was I thinking of, putting my very troubled body into the hands of such unknown unorthodoxy! But entering further, the pictures on the walls reassured me – large Gauguin prints, Monet, Van

*Sending Directions*

Gogh. And the reading matter in the waiting room was of immediate appeal.

The start of my first lesson was something I will never forget. A very slight, gentle-looking lady asked me to stand in front of a large wooden chair. This, I learnt later, had been Alexander's own teaching chair – and she was saying something about sitting down. Sitting down! Did she have any idea what pain that could start off without my doing a well-learned twist of my body, and a hand behind to steady me? At the same time, I somehow intuitively knew that such an option was not likely to be allowed. I don't remember much more except that she said very quietly, 'Just look a little up, out of that window,' and somehow, I have no idea how, I found myself sitting on the chair, feeling very calm, very easy, no pain anywhere and smiling with the sheer pleasure of it all.

From then on I wanted more and more and more. How did it work, and why? Would it help my feet which had often been painful since childhood? Migraines? So many questions. After a certain number of lessons, I pursued again the question of 'Would this help my feet as well as my back?' 'I don't see why not,' she said. No further elucidation, no further discussion about my feet – she didn't even look at them; just a persistent bringing me back to the present moment and F.M.'s verbal reminders to the neck, the head and the back. My teacher knew well that, only when she had gradually brought the primary arrangement of my neck and my head and my back more in order, would the feet cease to be a problem. So I began to forget about the feet and they were rarely mentioned again.

At a certain point I knew that she was going to start a small training course for teachers, and I kept thinking – I would really like to do this more than anything, not only for the ongoing help it had brought to my physical problems, but because it offered whole new horizons to be discovered about the relationship of the mind to the body, and so much else. Interests which I could foresee engaging me for the rest of my life. So one day, lying on her couch while she was working with me, I finally found the courage to ask if she would consider taking me on her next training course. To my great surprise she said, 'I've been hoping you would ask me that!', and from then on it all really began, in the autumn of 1955.

During the training, as a result of intensive Alexander work, deeply ingrained habits in the way one has used the body for many years are being touched and brought back to a better way of using the body. While at times this brings a great feeling of lightness and relief, at other moments the experience is one of profound exhaustion. Pupils have frequently remarked on a certain tiredness they have experienced later in the day after a lesson, and said, 'I can't believe it was the lesson, you hardly touched me!' Marjory said over and over again to us, 'Do less,' and I still think of that when working with a pupil. Whether it is to make a piece of pottery, engage with the supermarket, or whatever activity life presents at any given moment, by 'doing' less, so often the 'more' which we aspire to is actually realised.

During our first year of training it was all work on oneself. Learning to understand what Alexander meant by 'inhibition', or as Marjory put it to 'say no' to the immediate response or reaction to a stimulus, following with the messages without trying to do them, then to let the action take place and then to move on.

It was such a relief to be without judgement on what was already over, no 'Was that better?' or 'Now have I got it right?' Then there was work with the mirror – deciding on a specific movement, and then managing to 'inhibit' the very strong desire to change what didn't 'look' too good, and then to accept exactly what one saw, while continuing to work. Then the 'monkey' position. Alexander referred to this as 'the position of mechanical advantage' for the body. This led to 'hands over the back of a chair', added to the monkey position. 'Going up on the toes,' and so much more.

Marjory had some very descriptive images. One was when working with the arms. 'Imagine,' she would say, 'you have egg shells in your armpits. Too much pressure and the shells will break, too little, and the shells will fall out!' Another one she often used was to liken the head to a ping-pong ball playing on top of a fountain.

All this time my own use of my body and the whole shape of my body was changing.

One very clear example – in my teens, I longed for a strapless party dress, but my shoulder blades stuck out at the back in a way that no strapless dress could possibly accommodate and I had come to accept that this was the way I was made. Once, during my time on the training course, I was in a dress shop, trying on some dresses. At that time there were no cubicles, just a big room with mirrors all around. Idly looking at all the young women in various states of undress – as well as various misuses of bodies to my now-rather-interested Alexander eye, I noticed one girl and thought, 'Now she really has a good back, why couldn't mine have been like that?' On turning round to inspect her more closely, I discovered after some confusion that it was myself! When I went into the class the next morning I said to Marjory, 'What have you done with my sticking-out shoulder blades?' She smiled and said quietly, 'I wondered when you would notice.'

She never pushed, always waiting, watching for you to discover the next step for yourself. Toward the end of the first year we were introduced to placing the hands on the leg of a colleague lying on the couch. We also worked with a pot as a preparation for bringing the hands on to a pupil's head. All this was practice for the need to maintain the use of one's self, while receiving the very strong stimulus of working on another person's body. Eventually we were putting our hands on each other and learning to talk through the procedures before any action took place.

Another big step, during the third year of training, was to be asked, usually without warning, to go into the room to assist Dr Barlow by taking the head of a pupil who was on the couch while he worked on the rest of the pupil's body. For some years after training, I worked for a time as an assistant, which was a wonderful opportunity to consolidate what I had learned. I also had a teaching slot in the practice, which offered a great diversity of pupils and their problems.

A well-known Jungian therapist, a delightful lady, came in to her second lesson full of joy, saying 'I see! Alexander's "No" is not a negative – it's a positive!' She had many lessons until the end of her life and I felt privileged to be teaching her.

A young, sturdy, athletic chap who had badly damaged his back playing rugby and been through hospitalisation and much medical treatment was sent to Dr Barlow, who passed him on to me for lessons. He was in a great deal of pain with even small movements, and wore a corset most of the time. His real passion in life was to get back to playing rugby, and if the Alexander Technique seemed it might help, then he would work at it. And he did. After about a year, he was out of the corset, at home and at work, but still wore it when travelling on the underground – not a good place for back sufferers! Gradually the time between his lessons lengthened and then I didn't hear from him. After about a year a postcard came – 'I played my first game of rugby last week. All well. Thanks.'

Another gentleman was unknowingly the means of illustrating a principle I learnt from Marjory Barlow. He was slight in body but very stiff. He appeared very willing, came regularly, always punctual, but after a great many lessons, we seemed to be making no headway at all. I told my teacher I just didn't feel I could go on taking his money with such little visible change taking place. She said, 'If he keeps on coming, he is coming for something, but he may not know what it is. Don't turn him away.'

In a rather similar encounter I gave many lessons to a very pleasant woman who had problems which were helped, but never to the extent I would have wished for. Something was just not happening. One day she was on the table and I had been working quietly on her for a while when the words popped out of my mouth, 'When did you last have a good cry?' 'Cry!' she said, 'I never cry!' I said something like 'OK. That's alright.' When I took her up off the table, she burst into floods and floods of tears.

So I think one can never know, or assume to know anything about the person who has presented themselves to you. It is borne out by this final story of an elderly woman who had had a number of lessons, but would frequently phone and ask if I could see her that day, or at

## Sending Directions

least as soon as possible. At the end of one of these 'emergency' lessons she looked at me as if expecting something more and then said, 'But you haven't done what you usually do?' I thought, 'What is it that I have not done?' – no two lessons ever being quite alike. When I asked her, she indicated a vague sort of widening of her ribcage, and explained that the reason why she came for a lesson was that when her gall bladder flared up, 'This is the only thing that helps!'

In 1971, having sold our house well, we had sufficient savings so that when Adam lost his job it seemed a good moment for him to join a training course, something the head of training had long hoped he would be able to do.

By the early 1980s we felt the time had come for us to at last move out of London. Our daughter was at university and we had already been doing some teaching in West Sussex, and felt it could be a viable situation. We decided that to start a training course would be our next venture. Certainly to train a pupil to teach would be a further step in our own understanding of what Alexander taught.

We had many applications, partly because there were not nearly so many training courses at that time. We settled for ten pupils – but how to choose, and who could tell what changes might take place in someone with all that intensive work over a period of three years? Ideally, we were looking for people who had a real interest in Alexander's technique, who had read his books, had had a full course of lessons and wanted to take the adventure a step further.

One person we were very happy to be able to train, on our third training course, was our daughter, who, much to our surprise, asked us if we would consider taking her. We never pushed the Technique at her, but one way and another she had quite a lot of work from us. During her teenage years she began to have problems with a hip joint and then would often ask for lessons, but it never occurred to us that she might one day think of training. She now teaches at a well-known girls' school and also at a private college in London.

We brought our training course to an end in 1999. It had, for all of us I think, been a good experience, and many of our trainees are still in touch with us. Strong bonds are formed amidst all the inevitable ups and downs on such courses with the constant need to see and accept each others' difficulties over such a long period of time. A strong sense of humour can help.

Dr Barlow warned me that to spend one's life as an Alexander teacher 'will never make you rich – it is not an entrepreneurial profession – but it's a good life', and he hoped I would enjoy it as much as they had done. I think that this was exactly right and I am so grateful that life presented me with this opportunity, and that I have been able to commit myself to it for most of my life. I still enjoy teaching – no two people are alike, so the work never fails to be interesting.

In 1986, I was in my fifties and teaching the Alexander Technique both privately as well as training new teachers. I was also teaching part-time at a well-known music school. At that time little was known about osteoporosis – only that it was something which you really did not want to encounter, and not much talked about. And there was no internet available for research!

One day our local surgery was offering free tests and, wanting to know more, I took the test and was startled to be told I had full osteoporosis ( not even just osteopenia). I didn't believe the result, and had a private test done elsewhere – exactly the same result.

For a time I took the prescribed, large, chalky, calcium tablets, but I was very busy and happy in my life, and quickly forgot about this diagnosis. However, fast forwarding over the next thirty years, I now see in retrospect that this disease was steadily developing. I had about nine instances of cracked ribs. The doctor told me, 'There is no treatment – we don't strap people up any more – yes, you can drive – it will be painful for about three weeks. Take pain killers.'

Then there was an ankle fracture, and one leg in plaster for two months. Osteoporosis was never mentioned again, until two years ago, with an almost exact replica of the painful step onto the train at the very beginning of my story. Mounting a steep step in the street, pain such as I have never experienced ever, shot through my whole body. A scan showed fractures at lumbar vertebra 4, and thoracic vertebrae 9, 10 and 11, and a whole change in body shape, traumatic in itself!

Thinking back, I can only say how truly grateful I am now for all those many years when I was under such intensive Alexander Technique work, both on myself and with others. I am sure that kept me out of major trouble for such a long time, in the circumstances.

It was also very clear to me at the time that each of the minor rib fractures were the result of the inappropriate use of my body. One example – when sitting in a chair, I twisted sideways in order to lean over the arm of the chair, in order to pick a knitting needle up from the floor, INSTEAD of standing up and turning round in order to kneel down. This is a good example of what Alexander calls 'end-gaining': not attending to the means as to how you achieve your end.

And now, in my old age, I think very, very often of what Alexander is reported to have said in his later years when asked if he still practised the Technique which he had discovered. He replied that he 'wouldn't dare not to!' Perhaps that's one final lesson from F.M. to all of us!

## Gentle but Effective
Melody Hirst

In 2001, I had been attending a physiotherapy clinic for many years where I was being treated on a regular basis (sometimes three times a week when the pain was at its worst) regarding my multiple musculoskeletal dysfunctions, which according to the physiotherapist's report included:

> *Left and right sacroiliac joint*
> *Lumbar spine vertebrae L2–L4 facet joints*
> *Upper costovertebral joints of ribs one to eight*
> *Cervical spine and bilateral facet joint dysfunction*

The physiotherapist had said that she felt that, although I was a diligent patient and did all the exercises I was asked to do and I went swimming and tried to keep myself active, she did not think my body was responding as it should to physiotherapy and thought I should have a break.

Having fallen from a horse at age fourteen and landing awkwardly on my head, I had been suffering back pain since my early twenties. Pain became increasingly worse as I got older, especially after the birth of my two children. In my thirties I was also diagnosed with rheumatoid arthritis.

Having tried physiotherapy, osteopathy, reflexology, acupuncture and a chiropractor, and also endeavouring to keep active with swimming, walking and Tai Chi, I was finding that the spells of being able to lead a normal life between attending physiotherapy sessions were getting shorter. I seemed to be spending more and more time dealing with severe and debilitating pain, at best suffering some pain on a daily basis.

My lifestyle was becoming more and more restricted. Doing the things I really wanted to do was not a reality anymore.

*Sending Directions*

Having tried everything, I felt that I must be 'doing something wrong'. I had found some information about the Alexander Technique and friends persuaded me to try some lessons. My main thought at the time was, 'This is my last chance to try to get rid of the back pain'.

With an open mind I attended my first lesson. I hobbled in and walked out with less pain. What were my first impressions? Having experienced the rigours of physiotherapy and a chiropractor, I was struck by the gentleness of the Technique. No rough handling and no pain! And better still I didn't have to undress, something I had found very difficult in a physiotherapy session when doubled up in a great deal of pain!

From that first moment of experiencing 'hands on', it still amazes me how gentle but effective the Technique proves to be. I cannot describe adequately how I still feel when I lie in the semi-supine position. If for some reason I have to forego this at home I feel deprived!

It is a lovely memory for me, the first time I went on a long hill walk shortly after beginning the Alexander Technique. I followed my teacher's advice to remember 'head, neck and back' as I walked and to be conscious of my body throughout the walk. The joy the following morning was to find that I had not only enjoyed a pain-free walk, but had not damaged myself in any way and was not suffering any pain!

My other joyful memory is of holding my newborn grandson for the first time, knowing that I would be able to be 'an active and hands-on Grandma'. Seven years on, I never thought I would be playing football and tennis with him, but I do and it is tiredness, not excruciating pain, that results from the activity!

My lessons have changed my life. Yes, I still have times when my back can be a problem (it is usually when I have not remembered to be aware of my body and the Technique), but I now have the techniques at my finger tips to recover quickly, whereas before AT I would be restricted for months from any physical activities and there was always the fear that it could get worse! That fear has gone and been replaced with a much more positive outlook. AT has been life changing; it has also been life enhancing. I feel that, at nearly sixty-four, I am doing far more now than I did in my twenties!

Ten years on, I still look forward to my lessons and sometimes have to remind myself just what an incredible journey I have made and am still experiencing. I also realise how privileged I am to be able to continue with the Alexander Technique!

Thank you to the Alexander Technique and to my teacher for guiding me and giving me the opportunity to enjoy a full and active life without crippling pain.

# Memories in the Making
## Amie Shorey

Around thirty-two weeks into my pregnancy, everything had been going really well. One day I walked to get bread from our local deli and ended up getting a few more things. Carrying these bags and walking at my usual pace, I started to feel quite a bit of pain in my pelvis. I thought this would pass but over the next couple of days it actually felt worse. I realised that I had symphysis pubis dysfunction (SPD) and this was confirmed by my midwife. Everything I had read about SPD said that I would have to manage it very carefully, and that if it got worse I could end up using crutches, and might have to rethink my birth plan. Naturally I was very worried. At my next AT lesson I mentioned my pelvic pain. My teacher showed me a model of the pelvis and explained how the pain was caused. She taught me to add to my AT directions the thought: let the sacrum, the back of the pelvis, be free so that its two wings can move together at the front. Most important: I had to inhibit the temptation to let my weight fall on the sacrum. She took me into the 'monkey' position and taught me how to move and walk so as to manage the pain. This lesson was most useful; I followed these directions and thought as often as I could about my pelvis releasing at the back and moving together at the front.

To my amazement, the pain lessened significantly and I found myself even able to stand on one leg again and walk with more ease. To be on the safe side I kept up all my Alexander Technique awareness.

By the time I went into labour, the SPD had gone away completely. None of the stories or research I had read about SPD had said that this was a possibility, and yet it went away altogether for me. I am really grateful to my teacher for teaching me this aspect of the Alexander Technique, which enabled me to go on and have the birth I had wanted for my baby and also gave me greater comfort toward the end of my pregnancy.

On Saturday 21st January, I opted for a longer-than-usual lie-in to stock up on sleep as Maya's due date was on Thursday. It was a lovely, gentle, calm start to the day and we were very happy spending the time together. My husband Steve went to watch Queens Park Rangers play football at lunchtime and I was going to shop for dinner as we had his friend coming round that night. As Steve left, I had some twinges and felt strangely purposeful. I decided I ought to get to Marks & Spencer's quickly as I had a suspicion that labour could be close, but thought that would be too good to be true. When I got back I was keen to dust and clean frantically until I felt that I should get some rest. A couple of hours later I was getting contractions, so I rang Mum, as I had begun pacing the room and wanted to check with her if I was in labour. I rang Steve to warn him that labour could be imminent. Sure enough, it kept up momentum. At one point I was overcome with emotion at the thought of giving birth to Maya in the pool at the hospital and I started to cry with joy and excitement.

For the next few hours we used a TENS machine, and with each contraction we moved together as we had learnt from the AT teacher in a joint lesson we had toward the end of my pregnancy. Steve was very excited and hugely supportive, and kept me comfortable. We had the lighting down low and music on, and just spent time between 5 p.m. and 1.30 a.m.-ish together, handling contractions and staying calm. At one point my mood became anxious as I became too concerned with the interval between my contractions. I stopped monitoring this; Steve accurately prescribed me some homoeopathy and we got back on track as I calmed down again.

Around 1.30 a.m. contractions were very close together and very intense, so we gathered everything up for the car. As we were getting the final bits together, I told Steve, in quite an assertive way, that we had to leave immediately as the baby was coming! Steve got us to the hospital in twenty minutes: all the red lights turned green for us as we drove up to them and we got ourselves to triage amid contractions about two to three minutes apart.

Unfortunately when I was checked over, the midwife told me I was only two centimetres dilated, three centimetres during contractions. The pain was really intense and regular and I was very disheartened, as I wasn't sure I could cope with the rest of the labour at this pace. She

*Sending Directions*

also told us that she didn't know if there was a midwife qualified to let us use the birthing pool. I lost heart and started pleading with Steve for some sort of help. We used a homoeopathic remedy again, which restored my mood.

Luckily, we were allowed to stay at the hospital, as we lived too far away to go home. We were admitted into the birth-pool room. I got straight into the shower and felt the water to be much more effective than the TENS machine. The midwife pushed down on my lower back during contractions, which really helped; so Steve took over and helped aim the shower head at the pain. Contractions were very fast, with little time to rest in between. Steve was very good at passing me drinks, giving me encouragement and didn't stop his hard work for a moment. I felt really supported by him and we were both very focused – which is why I believe labour began to progress so quickly.

The midwife commented a few times on how relaxed my shoulders were during contractions, which I attribute to the Alexander Technique practice. After just one hour in the shower I was examined on the bed and given gas and air, which worked very well for me. I was told that I was between seven and eight centimetres dilated, which really lifted me, and after a few more contractions I was allowed into the pool. The gas and air gave me my sense of humour back and I was able to see some of the funny side of things. Steve was brilliant with encouraging words, kisses and hands-on help. The contractions continued for a while in the water with the beautiful playlist of music in the background that Steve had put together.

Soon I was told I could start pushing; the urge was really strong. The midwife placed a mirror underneath me and for the next twenty minutes I asked if I was crowning after each push, as Maya searched for the right way out. Little did I realise how lucky I was with the speed of this stage of labour until the midwife pointed this out to me – which also really lifted my spirits and gave me more encouragement.

I could hear the midwife singing along to some of our songs and this made me feel that she was on board with our birthing experience. Her name was Sarah, and she was about my age. She seemed totally competent and we had complete faith in her, so the environment around us was as I had wished it would be.

Suddenly the midwife told us that Maya had lots of dark hair. This surprised us and got us excited. Steve could see this in the mirror too. I started talking to Maya, encouraging her to come out. Not long after, the midwife told us that she would be out in a couple of pushes and Steve got really excited. The sensation of this was very strange and I was keen for the next contraction to start. When it did, I pushed hard for a couple more contractions. Then I felt Maya come out and into the water. We could see her in the pool and I started to sob with joy as she was handed to me.

The midwives asked me to blow on her face to encourage her to take her first breath. Steve looked on and was totally in awe. He cut the cord and Maya was put under the heat as she was a little blue. She was then passed back to me as I sat on the birthing stool. We were moved onto the bed where I could carry on feeding Maya and she was lovely and calm throughout. Later Steve held Maya and had skin to skin contact with her for a long time. It was an amazing memory-in-the-making for me to watch them fall in love.

The midwife told us that in five years she could only recall one other woman who had been as calm and collected during birth. This surprised me: I didn't realise I had been calm, as it had been so intense and we had been so focused throughout. She then gave us her home address and asked us to send a picture of Maya to her, as this was her ninty-eighth delivery and one she wanted to remember as it was so calm, and she said how much she enjoyed it. Other midwives came into the room and were surprised to see that Maya had already been born. It was as if they wanted to see for themselves that the labour had genuinely progressed that quickly. We took Maya home that evening. It felt so normal and natural to have Maya with us.

# The Beagler
Anonymous

At the age of about forty-five, I began to experience severe pain in both of my knees. After examination, I was told that I had damaged the cartilage in the knees. This damage had initially been caused by the use of a kicking strap on a sailing dinghy and made worse by many years of beagling, which involves running or trotting over ground that is very often rough, and causes the foot and knee to be out of alignment. I was advised to have physiotherapy and to wear a skiing support to reduce the strain on the knee. I did this for a couple of years, but the pain became an increasing problem. A scan revealed that I had arthritis in my right knee and torn cartilages in both my knees.

Over the following two years, I had four arthroscopies on my knees followed up by more physiotherapy. I was told to stop beagling or risk ending up in a wheelchair. I didn't take this advice, despite the pain becoming an increasingly severe problem and starting to have secondary consequences. Because of the knee problem, and without my realising it, I had started to change the way I walked and this caused problems with my back so that this also became painful. I found out that a slow walk through an art gallery or museum became very difficult to handle, and if I sat in a car for over two hours, it might take me five minutes to ease myself out of the car. I was also using a painkilling gel to make the situation more bearable.

It was at this stage, aged fifty-eight, that a friend of my wife suggested the Alexander Technique. At first I was very sceptical, but I had also reached the stage where I was ready to try virtually any means to solve the problem. I was given the name of a teacher who had trained as a doctor and also in the Alexander Technique. In an initial examination she explained, among other things, what the Technique involves and gave me a couple of books about the Technique. She also said that, although she had had considerable success teaching people with lower back pains, this would be the first time that she had had to deal with knee problems. I read the two books and decided to go ahead with a series of lessons; in part this was because I didn't have many options left, but also because the risks attached to trying out the Technique are so low. No medicaments, no surgery – and moderate costs. Following her advice, I booked for a fairly intensive series of two or three lessons a week at the beginning, with the intention of reducing this once I had made a beginning. Much to my surprise and enormous pleasure – I started feeling the benefits of using the Technique after a very short time.

A few weeks after my first lesson, I had gone out beagling, but only walking, not running or trotting. I was not wearing my knee ski support and had not taken any pain killers. Some hounds had separated from the main pack and the Master asked a friend to go and bring them back. As the friend ran past me, he called out and asked me to accompany him in order to help. I took a deep breath, thought to myself that I would take the risk, directing as instructed, and ran after him. I was amazed that I could run without any pain whatsoever, either immediately or later on – especially in bed at night. My back pain had also almost completely disappeared although it remained a small problem for a while. If the pain recurred, I would almost immediately find somewhere where I could lie down to apply the Technique; friends and colleagues quickly became accustomed to seeing me doing this. It is now many years since I last had back pain.

I am now seventy-three years old and still go out beagling two or three days a week (more often three than two). But I stick to the rule of always applying my directions before starting to run. These days, my running speed is probably not much faster than the fast walking pace of many of my younger companions. But I happily accept that as a consequence of the age difference. The point is that, twenty-six years after I was told to stop beagling or risk ending up in a wheelchair, I am still running without pain and without painkillers. I find it essential to do my lying down very regularly and continue to have lessons about once a month. I am still making progress and my long-established stoop (postural thoracic kyphosis) is beginning to straighten out. Sometimes people say that, surely by now I have learnt how to use the Technique. Perhaps so. But I remember that George Bernard Shaw, who was introduced to the Technique in his eighties, was asked the same question, he said that he could not afford to take the risk of not continuing with his lessons. I feel the same way.

# The Primary Control of the Use of the Self

> *The experiences which followed my awareness of this were forerunners of a recognition of that relativity in the use of the head, neck, and other parts which proved to be a primary control of the general use of the self. (The Use of the Self, 1946, p. 9)*

In Alexander's work, the central organisational law of this complex system of ours is the relationship between our head, neck and back – the primary command or 'control' we share with all other vertebrates which 'is indirectly responsible' for the 'working of all the other parts of the organism'. (*The Universal Constant in Living*, p. 161) When we don't interfere with this central command, the control of our complex organism is rendered comparatively simple. Yet, judging by the stories in this book, not interfering with it is far from easy, for how we use it is inextricably bound up with how we mentally respond to what is going on in our lives.

Veronica Pollard's story reinforces this when, having graduated as an Alexander Technique teacher, she talks about a long bicycle trip that she undertakes and finds on it 'the poise of my head in relation with my body in movement, really was the key to freedom and ease of motion!' As David Green finds with his teacher, for most this primary relationship is central to Alexander Technique lessons from the beginning: 'Early on my teacher introduced the idea of "primary control" and the relationship between neck, head and back.' Initially sceptical, Geraldeen Fitzgerald perseveres and finally perceives results from her changes in thought as well as her physical habits. At that point, she says, 'I imbibed this perception and began to use the AT to change the poor habitual use of my head, neck and back, which was producing the back pain to begin with.'

A virtuous circle begins with the thought of allowing the neck to be free, so that the head can go forward and up, and the back can lengthen and widen. It is, in Helen May's words earlier in this book, 'a life sentence after all, one that I welcome, one that I enjoy'.

## The Wheel Comes Full Circle
### Veronica Pollard

I have had a love affair with the bicycle since I was six and was given a shiny red one for Christmas. Later, like most teenage girls, I lost interest, partly because I lived in one of the hilliest cities in England where the bus tickets cost pennies. But when I came to Bristol to go to university, the accommodation was a couple of miles away from the lecture halls. So I bought a bike and fell back in love with cycling.

Spool forward a few years and, although I still loved cycling, I was getting tension headaches, neck aches and shoulder aches when I did a day's ride. First I looked at the bike set up, then I asked other people if they had the same result, and was told that they didn't, or at least not to the extent that I did. At some point someone mentioned the Alexander Technique. I heard them, but I didn't know what it was: it was probably too expensive, too weird and thus not for me.

Then I heard that there was a drop-in AT class that cost very little at a local dance studio. I dropped in and was amazed at the difference the teacher's hands-on made to my aching shoulders and neck. After a few evenings I asked her about the cycling issue. She suggested that I bring my bike in the next week. I did and, having got some of the other students to hold it up, she asked me to show her how I would cycle. I remember what I did very clearly. I squashed myself down by forcing my head back and down and raised my shoulders. I could feel the arc of pain I got when cycling. We all laughed. The teacher showed me that I didn't need to do any of that to cycle and introduced me (and the rest of the class) to the idea of moving in a very different way. I was pretty much hooked at that point and within a few months had started to train as a teacher. I had more bike lessons, sitting lessons, other activity lessons and gradually got better at riding my bike, as well as at just about everything else. My life was getting easier and calmer, and I had changed a lot of my poor thinking and bad ideas.

In fact I pretty much forgot about how painful cycling had been and signed up for a cycle trip from Land's End to John o'Groats without a second thought. This was in 2007, which was four years after I'd finished my AT teacher training.

LEJoG, or 'the End to End' as it's called, is one of the world's iconic cycle rides, going from the most southerly point to the most northerly point of Britain. Our route was going to be about 970 miles and we were going to take two weeks without a break.

I started training and by the time the group met up in Penzance, I was feeling confident that I was fit enough to do the trip. The first couple of days were difficult – the hills of Cornwall and Devon are numerous and steep, and I got a bit of backache. But from then on, with an average of seventy-five miles a day, I didn't get a single ache anywhere. I also had lots of time to think about what I was doing with myself while cycling, and I started to notice things that I could change or stop. I stopped squashing down a bit when I started to go uphill and found I had more energy to put in my legs – a far more useful place. I could really see that all I needed to do was, in essence, sit down and move my legs. If I came forward from my hips I could reach the handlebars without using my shoulders and I didn't need to grip the bars any more than necessary to keep my hands on them. Oh, and the poise of my head in relation with my body in movement, really was the key to freedom and ease of motion!

I now get quite a few students who want to improve how they ride their bikes. I am happy to show them how to do it differently and with less effort, combining the two things I love – teaching the Alexander Technique and cycling.

# The Real Deal
David Green

I like to write, and am pleased to share my Alexander story. I like to think of writing as being, to some degree, a reflection of the mind. I can come back and read the stuff later and think 'that's nice' or 'that's right', or maybe just 'that's a load of rubbish' and chuck it in the bin. Spontaneity in writing captures the moment; it's our take on events at a particular time and depends somewhat on what's coming through the senses. And what comes through the senses affects our mental and physical comportment. My Alexander teacher quite often homes in on this aspect of the Technique during a lesson, providing insight into the psychophysical world in which we live, easily borne out by observation of ourselves and others.

Spontaneous writing is also a good barometer for inner reflection, warts and all. A different mood brings a different perspective. Early judgements may be toned down and premature ego-based musings proven groundless. Occasionally though, things on the page come together and are worth keeping. It's not really the subject matter that counts here, it's the way we address it; it's how we bring ourselves to the table. We have a degree of duty to ourselves to do things right. Later, when reading my own stuff, I will often have developed a slightly different take on the subject. Nothing is totally fixed; we move on and the mind is always tweaking and updating itself with new experiences.

Writing inhibits the constant backroom chatter where the mind loves to hang out, and directs us to a blank sheet where we can begin our stories and ideas. It's a great accompaniment for the Alexander student. The mind is slowed down to the pace of the pen and given a break from the mental humdrum to which it has been accustomed. I like to write down ideas and observations and discuss them with my teacher during the next Alexander lesson; not exactly homework, but a bit of an effort to describe how I might have perceived and made use of my previous lesson. It also lets me begin a dialogue with my Alexander teacher, and leads on to discussions on different aspects of the Technique. I quietly anticipate my Alexander lessons and meeting up with my teacher; I gain a tremendous amount from this relationship. So here's to my teacher and friend.

At the beginning of my second Alexander lesson my teacher looked at me and asked pleasantly, 'Do you think this is a load of rubbish?'

Over the following day or so, after some head scratching, I concluded that this was such a great question. It embodied the teacher's confidence in herself and her profession. There was an implied 'Come on board for the journey; I'll be there, but the choice is entirely yours'.

Only lesson two, and I was looking forward to the next one. I already wanted to be where my teacher was. First impressions do count, and I was certainly impressed. My teacher has natural poise and a grace from times long gone. Movement, awareness and connection combined into a single action, the like of which I was seeing for the first time. I felt welcome, comfortable and at home. She has patience and commitment, and the defensive barriers I normally employ in any new situation soon began to slip away. It would be hard to imagine a better beginning for a student. In percentage terms, if I ever achieve just five percent of what my teacher already has, I'll be a very happy chap. It goes without saying that I bought a season ticket and I've just renewed it!

So here was and still is the first and most important insight of my Alexander journey. My teacher mirrors her profession perfectly, she is the quintessential exponent of the Alexander Technique, the perfect fusion of mind and body – the real deal – absolutely no question.

A good few years ago I was on the beach after a day's work in the far north of Scotland. Vastly overweight, with a twenty-five-a-day cigarette addiction and alcohol making up a large part of my social life, I was not the nimblest of people on the beach that evening. From a distance I might have been mistaken for some marine life washed up with the last tide. Still, life wasn't too bad. I could pretty well do what I wanted, go where I wanted, and eat and drink what I wanted. Until, that is, I slipped on a shiny little rock and life was never the same again.

## The Primary Control of the Use of the Self

In the early hours the following morning I awoke with lower-back pain the like of which I would not wish on anyone. (Well, almost anyone, I'm no saint!) The period between waking and the receptionist arriving at work at 6 a.m. can only be described as survival.

That morning I swore that if I did survive the day intact, things would definitely change; but for now it was still today and I had this thing to which my head was attached, and it continued through my body and somehow fixed onto my legs. It was my spine and it didn't work any more; it sent excruciating pain in uncontrolled spasms into my pelvis and legs. Maybe it needed treating with a little more respect. Spines are important, I thought, and I promised mine that for the rest of its natural life I would be the picture of kindness toward it.

My first promise was to relieve it of the forty pounds of excess flab that hung over my trouser belt, and that promise I did manage to keep. Eventually I did kick my love affair with alcohol and nicotine but, for now, there was still the pain, and men and pain do not go together, believe me! Childbirth is said to be even more painful. Well, I'm not too sure about that! My wife has had two children and I was present at both births – so I know about these things!

Later that morning a very nice doctor gave me an injection in the backside. The pain slipped away and I was back in the land of the living. He also phoned his friend down the road, a physiotherapist who saw me out of hours and, after some worrying manipulation of my back and legs, I emerged onto the street more or less intact, carrying strict instructions to seek further attention should things get worse.

Things never did go back to that painful day, but my back was never really the same again. I began calling myself 'old glass back'. I seemed to 'pull it' all the time and I was visiting a physiotherapist with increasing regularity.

One day, local intelligence pointed me to a particular physiotherapist. Bad backs were the speciality. The tip was right, and this last physiotherapist, while doing an excellent job on my back, also suggested that I try some preventative therapy. She said I might try some lessons in the Alexander Technique. I had every reason to listen to her – she had fixed my back again – and so, despite never having heard of the Alexander Technique, I booked my first lesson. Definitely the right decision, absolutely no question.

I remember beginning my first lesson a little tense and defensive, but not unduly worried. I had never heard of the Alexander Technique before, save for the leaflet I'd got from my physiotherapist. The leaflet suggested to wear loose clothing but nothing much else that I remembered. I had entertained myself with the thought of some kind of head or body massage, which I must admit posed no undue trepidations for me!

With hindsight I can see how difficult it must be for the Alexander teacher. There I was, bent forward, leaning on my elbow across the desk looking confidently bemused! Forty-five years of amassing a vast armoury of habitual responses culminating in a permanent back problem, and now here I was sitting opposite my new teacher. As I've said (and I make no apologies for repeating it) my teacher was the model which got me beyond the first couple of lessons. She had made an immediate impact on me and I was keen to learn more, although my understanding of what 'learning' meant in relation to the Alexander Technique was a completely incorrect one when I began. I needed to begin to unlearn what I thought was the right way to use myself, and this was my teacher's job, although I was blissfully unaware of the challenge ahead of her at the time.

Early on, my teacher introduced the idea of 'primary control' and the relationship between neck, head and back. She gave me a slip of paper on which she'd written, 'Let the neck be free, so the head can go forward and up, and the back lengthen and widen'.

My first reaction was to check the handwriting style; I don't know quite why, I just did that sort of thing in those days! Closer to the truth maybe was that I just noticed the style; it was nice and flowing and easy on the eye; no surprises there then!

## The Primary Control of the Use of the Self

I brought some real concentration to that piece of paper over the next few weeks. I pulled it from my wallet regularly until it became more of a mantra. I was beginning something and I was keen to learn. I don't think this did me any harm; rather I was beginning subconsciously to build on the trust and perspectives my teacher was passing on. I think we need to nurture this inner feeling of wanting to progress as a whole person. Perhaps it's a bit similar to yearning for a long-lost friend; but in our case our real self is not lost forever; he's just around the corner and when we do meet up, it's handshakes and smiles all round! It's not end-gaining, which is a bit ego-based and selfish; it's the correct direction to focus the mind. To become a truly wholesome person is surely the way forward for everyone.

My early understanding of the idea of the whole person was probably too much of an intellectual concept. I've seen dozens of books on the shelves of WH Smith and read similar material, but still from a distance, from just an intellectual stand point. While working with my teacher on my own use, and homing in on my own tensions in my body and mind, I slowly began to appreciate that each bit of it is interdependent. Even better was the realisation that the mind and intellect are inextricably linked to the physical bits. It seems quite extraordinary now to have thought otherwise. God knows how many pointers my teacher gave me in the process of attaining this insight. Somewhere else in the mix there are our emotions, the good ones and the bad ones. I often (and still do sometimes) confused negative emotions with rational thinking. It gets you nowhere, believe me.

My teacher has often explained that our physical self is bound to suffer if we are continually engaging in negative mental and emotional misuse. As a result, we can easily adopt a poor and withdrawn demeanour: chin down, drooping shoulders, or maybe an aggressive 'what the ...' attitude. A quasi-zombie like existence which, if we don't watch it, becomes the norm. There are millions of people walking around in varying degrees of this twilight world. No wonder we have wars and world instability.

I'll be quite open about it. Now I choose not to be unhappy. I can choose not to go to places which make me emotionally insecure. I don't mean emotion doesn't have its place; it does and I have genuine compassion for people on the planet who have such dreadful lives to put up with. Thinking of people who are regularly faced without the basics for human survival is making me feel a little emotional at this moment, and it is the correct response to this kind of reflection.

How do I sit this kind of mental use and thinking along with F.M. Alexander's? Easily. I have a duty to organise my own use properly, both mentally and physically. To achieve this I need good primary control and an appreciation of the workings of the whole self. I will then have the opportunity to engage properly with the rest of the outside world. So I did make choices. First of all, as I said, I have chosen, with proper balance, not to be unhappy. I have made choices under my teacher's guidance to bring about the correct use of my own self, mental and physical, and have reaped the benefits. Choice is the main tool in my Alexander toolkit, which my teacher has freely given me. We all need to choose the correct use of ourselves. Get ourselves right and we can enjoy the journey.

I have seen some remarkable and welcome changes in myself since I met up with my teacher. I do not have a back problem, my back has actually become stronger and so have my legs. My back has regained much of the lost space and territory it used to own. Neither have I been troubled with my dodgy shoulder. I breathe better and may claim better vision and hearing. Most of all though, and this has only started to kick in over the last few months, I feel much happier. I wasn't unhappy before and that may seem like a contradiction but it's not. I have just chosen not to visit those places which from time to time can make me periodically unhappy. I don't need to engage in conflict, suffer from road rage or hold unhealthy opinions regarding politics or the world at large.

Even more importantly, we have to accept where we are: we cannot have everything, and sometimes we have to be happy with our own lot, with the bed that we have constructed. It's not necessarily better on the other side of the fence. In other words, one has to choose not to give in to feelings of insecurity which, when looked at closely, are almost certainly baseless. Just like a marriage, we have to work on

## The Primary Control of the Use of the Self

ourselves to find the real peace and harmony within us which we all seek. To me that's something basic F.M. Alexander was telling us. It's perfectly legal to choose not to be unhappy or not to misuse our backs and necks. Yes, we can all choose to have a choice. Not my words; I've read that somewhere else. It's truth, though, will set us all free.

Be breathed, be seen, be heard, be tasted, be well-used, be aware and be connected. Doesn't that sound awesome! But few of us understand it.

It's also important not to take life too seriously. Go for a drink or two with a pal. Chew the fat. Sort out the world over a pint; it's all good stuff, it makes us tick. Go home and tell the wife that 'things are gunna change around here!' Well, maybe not the last bit, she might take me up on it and I am pushing fifty! Dust off the Triumph Bonneville in the corner of the garage and let the wind rush through the holes! Chill, as they say.

Let me expand a bit more on those early lessons. I have done a lot of work in front of the chair with my Alexander teacher. I enjoy it just as much now as the early days. On my first lesson though, as I mentioned earlier, after introductions, I sat down and sprawled out over the desk next to me and lent on my elbow, totally unaware of the message that sent out to my brand-new teacher. Which is such a strange thing. What I thought was quite well-mannered and fairly cool for a new occasion looked quite different from the other side of the desk. There were no wrong intentions; it was just a complete misconception of what I thought I was doing. With hindsight it definitely didn't look balanced in any shape or form; neither was it particularly polite.

That left my teacher with few alternatives. A few well chosen words, and I was sitting bolt upright! I now know that what I thought was a pretty good sitting posture was in fact quite the opposite. This was only just a start. I was still wound up like a spring. with tension from head to foot.

Under her guidance I began standing and sitting, and repeating this again. I began to realise I was using this spring inside me to complete the movement. My brain was saying 'ready, steady, here we go, blast off'! Neck and chin disappear, elbows thrust back, back bends and legs attempt to push the floor down to the next level! The result was not very pretty, and with the landing, I just managed to secure one side of my backside to the chair. Or was she moving the chair to stop my rear end from completely crash landing? What was wrong with me?

With a truly remarkable touch my teacher used her hands on my neck and back to dissipate the tension and re-establish the spinal link between head and pelvis. She encouraged me to think of my 'up'; 'keep thinking up'. She let me understand that I could stand when I wanted: it was my choice how and when to stand and sit. I began to realise there was no need to bring this agenda of tension and wasted energy to the simple act of standing and sitting. I began to enjoy this simple process using the minimum of effort: a big breakthrough, a big insight, and highly rewarding. I do like the interval between standing and sitting with a neck free from tension and connected to the lower back. When do I feel awkward and tense, wherever I am, I can go back and let my neck be free; just free; nowhere in particular; it already knows where to go; I don't need to tell it.

It's the same on my walks: too much interference is unhelpful. I like to be just aware of a freed-up neck, and the rest falls into place, especially the relaxed connection cascading down and releasing in the lower back, then all the way down to the feet. Breathing becomes natural and pleasantly unnoticed, fitting in with my walking pattern. Fictitious mental layers of self-importance dissolve and the senses zoom in to their real friends. I am not separate from anything or anyone anymore. It's just me, just David, some trees and a meandering brook.

I like working with the chair because it covers just about everything. My sitting bones know exactly where to go. My neck and shoulders release into my back and my weight flows through the sitting bones and out the chair legs down into the centre of the earth. When I stand I can see the lovely hills outside, and my peripheral vision takes in the rest of the room. I know my teacher is behind me. The space is nice.

I was at a concert in Manchester last week and pre-booked my ticket with care. Being tall, I didn't want to feel uncomfortable for the two-and-a-half-hour duration. But I was fine, no different to being in my Alexander chair. If a bit of tension started to appear, back to basics and let the neck free up; the rest falls into place. With no cramped-up bum and no aching neck and back, I was left to enjoy the show completely at ease; a stark contrast to my previous existence as 'old glass back'.

Very early on my teacher brought me up to speed with the importance of the lying down position, AKA semi-supine. I like incorporating some lengthening imagery centred around my breathing, but I do this while keeping my thoughts 'high', rather than direct concentration around my specific body bits. Sometimes I bring my attention on to my left hand and think about lifting it; instead I lift my right leg and carry on with this in various combinations. I may spend a full minute bringing attention to my hand then just pretend to lift it. The hand hasn't moved but there is a lot of background tension just waiting to jump in. It brings me close to what's actually going on and more aware of being able to choose what I decide to do, not jump straight into the action. Maybe I'll make a good poker player someday! If I'm too whacked after a long day and fall asleep I don't worry too much; my spine has rested and I can always start again later.

I don't pretend to know much about the brain or how it works. All that I need to know for now anyway is basically what I've been taught, especially when doing chair work. In the beginning I was wound up before I even began to stand. I knew I was going to be asked to stand so I had adopted this tense, wound-up posture in readiness for take-off. Why was I so keen to impress my teacher that I was the best person around when it came to standing up from a chair? Why had all this unnecessary extra preparation and energy been introduced before I had even decided to stand? Why did I want to finish standing before I even began the process?

I'm sure there will be a reason somewhere buried deep in my subconscious, but the point is, there is absolutely no need for it. I'm only standing up and sitting down, for Pete's sake! Time and again she encouraged me to not respond to these initial stimuli, which would rush in preventing the correct response. I didn't quite 'get it' in the early days but she persevered, using hand contact on my neck (how did she find it hidden away in my chest?) and back until eventually the penny started to drop, and I began slowly to ignore these ingrained habitual responses and choose, in my own time, a more rational response to the simple decision to stand up.

That's the trick for me. Time and bad use have created many incorrect responses. I need to stick to a process of inhibiting these and then directing my attention to the idea of the job in hand. Then I can proceed with how and when I begin the job. It's important for me to make this clear. There are no mysteries; it's a very practical and methodical way to use ourselves best. That's my take on this, and it works well for me. It's never too late in any situation; if I do allow all these bad responses into my thinking, I just slam the door shut. It doesn't matter; I've seen and heard them all before. I move my attention away quietly to the job in hand and I'm back where I should be. Simple.

My teacher often lifts my arms to help with the inhibition process, and still, occasionally, I try and give her some help. It's a spontaneous reaction but it's a good reminder that I need to decide what I need to accomplish; the old habitual responses don't work anymore.

When it came to the actual moment of standing, I had ditched my normal forty-five-year-old approach. What choices did I have, though? Perhaps a growing awareness that I only need place my attention on the simple idea of standing; my body would do the rest; I don't need anything else. I had help with the introduction of visual conceptions, and I always had the benefit of my teacher's 'think of your up'.

I mentioned early on to her that, as a substitute for stopping smoking and drinking and as a way to relax, I had gone back to the guitar, which I had abandoned decades earlier like so many others. I began putting a lot of effort into music theory so I could 'talk the talk' with keys and chords and begin with a more generic approach. Previous methods attempted in my younger days had delivered little. I have also put in a lot of practice and I'm beginning to have some fun. When I began my Alexander lessons I mentioned all this to my teacher. I also

*The Primary Control of the Use of the Self*

explained to her that although I could happily play a few simple pieces in private in my own company, playing in front of anyone was a very different matter. I could not even record myself on my own mobile phone!

Well, she said, bring the guitar in with you next time!

Why did I mention it? I must be mad, I thought, I can never do this. No alternative, though, and next time I brought the guitar with me. I tried to play it but I was holding so much tension when I started that I just went faster and faster, missed a lot of notes and finished on a low.

She explained head-on that this approach was classical Alexander and that he had coined the word 'end-gaining' to explain it. I wanted to get a result before I had even considered the implications involved to achieve it. I had never considered my own use! She reminded me of the importance of inhibiting habitual responses. 'Give the guitar some space; bring your attention to this lovely, spacious room for a moment and then, when you are ready, try something simple. Don't attack the guitar; bring your own way to it. Start afresh with a more reasonable approach, forget the need to finish and proceed at your own pace when you decide'. She was right, of course.

My misuse of the guitar mirrored the same misuse of myself. The good news now is both of us are well and truly in the recovery room. I have left behind the old habits that have caused me so much misuse in the past. I'd like to continue as an Alexander student for some time yet, and check in for a lesson every couple of weeks. I like my lessons, I like the Alexander Technique and most of all I like and respect my teacher and friend, simply the best. Absolutely no question.

## Leaving the Feet Behind
Kerry Downes

I am eighty. One afternoon nearly thirty years ago I was working at home and, by chance, saw most of a long television interview with Wilfred Barlow about the Technique; as a result I bought and read his book, The Alexander Principle. But it all seemed very complicated – a common reaction to new ideas – and I did nothing about it until 1995, when I found that singing hymns in church gave me a catch in the throat that brought tears to my eyes. Understanding that Alexander had started with a voice problem, I accepted a local offer of a trial lesson.

At the end of half an hour I had discovered that I habitually stood with my knees locked, and that this was quite unnecessary. From then on, with the exception of 'hands on the chair back', which I never made my peace with, the Technique seemed not complicated, but simple and entirely sensible. In the course of six years of lessons, the catch in the throat was never addressed directly, but within a few weeks two things in particular happened. Firstly, the recurrent headaches I had had for fifty years ceased, through changes in head and neck use. Secondly, one day in church, as the organist introduced a hymn I said to myself, 'I am not going to sing' – and sang the hymn without any trouble. I had not solved the problem, and it remained with me. But it now had two distinct components: firstly, whatever I was doing (but could not identify) that caught my throat, and secondly, the fact that actually singing while telling myself not to sing is rather a tall order. But I learned many things from my teacher, and became an Associate Member of an organisation for Alexander Technique teachers. And I began to learn things on my own.

I have always been interested in the way the body and the mind work, both generally and particularly in respect of our perception of the outside world and its pictures. I made some discoveries that were very small steps for mankind, but great leaps for me. In public I had never known what to do with my hands since the day I was told as a small child to take them out of my pockets. The answer was, of course, nothing. If there is no work for them to do such as holding or carrying, using tools, shaking hands with someone, or gesturing, let them hang loose at the ends of relaxed arms until wanted. Watching people in art galleries, I noticed that most of them, like me, adopted an attitude to look at the works on show. Now I found that by giving directions I could avoid that peculiar malaise known as 'museum feet'. I believe, in addition, that the thoughtful inhibition – I am not going to strike an attitude – removed a half-conscious-but-distracting sense of confrontation, and left me more comfortably aware both of my self and of the objects I had come to look at.

As an art historian, I am used to looking up at painted or elaborately plastered ceilings, hammerbeam roofs, or the tops of towers. One day it struck me that there are two ways of doing this: the thoughtless way and the thoughtful way. The thoughtless way involves lifting the head upwards and backwards, pulling all the cervical vertebrae into a backward arc that is possible but not congenial – literally craning the neck. This is very quickly tiring. The thoughtful way begins with the head at the very top of the spine: letting the spine be, all the way up, and moving the cranium only. If you still can't see high enough, moving the eyes up in their sockets will give another forty degrees or so of elevation, and no competent ceiling painter requires you to look above seventy degrees in all.

I also changed my driving style. Armchair travel has always seemed to me inappropriate for anyone in charge of a vehicle, and in fact the seats in coaches, buses and trains usually oblige the passenger to sit erect rather than lounge as so many car drivers do – although the reason has more to do with saving space than supporting spines. After a car service, I usually find that the mechanic has inclined the seat to drive it around the block. However, for many years I had put my hands on the wheel at the ten-to-two position, as this was said to give 'the best control', or at least the feeling of control. But I had thought about my back and my hands, not about my shoulders and arms. If for no other reason than reducing the distance I had to lift my arms, I found that hands at a quarter-to and quarter-past three meant less work for equal control and security.

Further discoveries occurred after I had stopped having lessons. A bug that once circulated in my system and lodged in my ear canals did some permanent damage to my balance, but we oldies are proverbially in danger of falling anyway. Out of doors a walking-stick (at the ready, not as a prop or an extra leg) may be helpful, but experience has shown that the only real defence against tripping, or slipping on ice, is constant vigilance: not only body awareness but also ground awareness. Loss of balance, however, is more insidious. The rolling heave of the old sailor is, if inelegant and laborious, a natural response to the fact that, with our feet together or proceeding along a narrow line, our top-heavy design becomes precarious as soon as the very delicate coordination of limbs, reflexes, eyes and inner ears is disturbed. One cannot roll splay-legged between the cabbage plants or the boxes in the utility room, or when crossing and turning in the kitchen while preparing a meal. A lot of domestic falls result from turning the head and torso suddenly and leaving the feet behind. Once you start to totter, a stiffening reflex operates in a supreme effort not to fall. Indeed, an expert wrote a few years ago in Statnews that this reflex was necessary and inevitable.

It is neither. In that precise moment of imbalance it is possible to say 'No': to go into 'monkey', letting the knees bend and the hips bend. Everything softens, but you are still on your feet, having allowed your centre of gravity to right itself.

And so, lastly, back to the throat problem. One Sunday as I stood up to sing I recalled a lesson on the 'Whispered Ah' in which the instruction was to think of that almost silent sound as being heard not by the teacher in front of me but by an imaginary person some way behind me. As the 'Ah' was not physically projected backwards but only thought of, no work was involved. What would happen if I thought of my singing voice reaching someone three rows behind me? It was a revelation. And then for the first time I understood the nature of my problem. It was rather like the attitude in the art gallery. In order to sing, I had thought of producing the voice (a cliché among singing teachers), of making a sound and projecting it out and forwards, instead of letting the sound come out. In other words, a lot of 'doing' with the throat muscles and also with the upper spine, which is very close indeed to the larynx. The tension was literally choking me.

It worked, and it still works. Moreover, it has worked long and well enough for me to begin thinking once more, safely, about the quality of the sound.

I have not finished learning yet.

# The Alexander Technique - My Personal Story
Geraldeen Fitzgerald

Until several years ago, my back pain was constant and my quality of life had deteriorated to the point of not being able to travel, having to wear an orthopaedic corset, and taking heavy painkillers that were also detrimental to my appetite and zest for life. I was dragging myself to work and home again, and every weekend I lay flat on my back, trying to recuperate for the next week's work.

I tried the Alexander Technique at one point, but stopped after six lessons because I sought an immediate solution to my problem. I later had significant improvements (decreased pain) with an osteopath, and then with a chiropractor and a physiotherapist. But only short term. Today I know that the Alexander Technique is a long-term solution, it's the 'patient' (the AT pupil) who works on her poor habitual use. Use?? Yes – the use of her body: her neck, limbs, head, spine – and of her mind. Because her mind, if willing and instructed, can interrupt bad habits. All those who have given up smoking tobacco understand.

If I finally decided to resume Alexander Technique lessons in 2003, it was because I met a colleague's husband at a business dinner. He was the only one at a table of eight (average age forty-five) who was not slouching. At the time I was using an ergonomic cushion on the restaurant chair for back support. Seeing this, he suggested that I try the AT. I said I already had. He said 'Try again. My back pain has gone. Even my golf swing has improved. So has my muscle tone.' He was roughly my age, but looked more fluid and fitter than I either looked or felt. So I retried the AT. He said, 'Persevere this time.' I promised him and myself that I would take a minimum of ten lessons.

I did not like my AT lessons any better the second time around: I got up and sat down for half of the lesson; the only good part was the second half, where I got to lie down (in the AT 'semi-supine position') after my hard work in the first part of the lesson. But I realised why my colleague's husband had specified 'ten lessons minimum' because, on the eighth lesson, I started to understand that my habitual use was dis-coordinating my body instead of coordinating it. I discovered (to my initial dismay) that in the Alexander Technique there is no concept of a right position for the body. Instead, the AT concentrates on promoting 'right direction', which must be learned anew because we have lost the sense of it. And most importantly, F.M. Alexander found that by changing our ways of thinking, we can free ourselves from physical misuse. In his own words, 'We can throw away the habits of a lifetime if we use our brains.'

The Alexander Technique is teaching me just that: how to change the habit of a lifetime. I was always 'shortening' my spine (slouching) instead of allowing it to lengthen. To recount, not the end of my story, for I am only in its middle myself, my scoliosis has 'evened out' and is no longer flagrantly visible. It doesn't impose itself any more on my daily feelings and sensations. My Alexander teacher explained to me what her own teacher had once said: 'People think that there is a body with a spine somewhere inside it. But you must learn that you have a spine with a body around it!'

I imbibed this perception and began to use the AT to change the poor habitual use of my head, neck and back, which was producing the back pain to begin with. I say the AT phrase, 'Let the neck be free, to let the head move forward and up, to lengthen and widen the back.' With ongoing lessons, understanding and attention on my part, my back has started to lengthen and widen more frequently and more generously. From a pitiful condition of weakness and vulnerability, it has become stronger and more resilient. My spine has untwisted itself to a significant extent, and has recovered its indispensable natural curves.

Today I am no longer afraid of pain, and it no longer dictates my life. Corsets and special cushions are things of the past. I can drive a car for a two-hour stretch, can sit in a train for a seven-hour journey to Italy, can do everything that pain – or the fear of it – had stopped me from doing. No more back pain. And I have noticeable flexibility and fluidity. One example: I get out of a sports car easily. Another: I get up elegantly from a low sofa without having to 'hoist' myself up. (Watch your colleagues or friends, or even twenty-year-olds hoist themselves out of low cars and low chairs!) I have a life again, with a well-rounded social, leisure and working schedule.

In the novel *The Cookbook Collector*, the writer describes back pain (p. 125):

> *The commute was bad enough. One morning he could not get out of bed. If he lay perfectly still, he felt no pain, but the moment he shifted his weight, his muscles seized up again. 'Barbara,' he called out, 'I can't move.' After three months, he had come to think of it as the pain – not his pain, but a larger, impersonal force. Everyone gave Mel advice. Dave recommended a chiropractor. Jonathan suggested that he hit the gym. 'I think,' Barbara said cautiously, 'you might want to talk to Rabbi Zylberfenig. Everybody had a guru. Even Sorel Fisher, his newest hire, insisted, 'I'll give you the name of my Alexander teacher.'*

And, in art imitating life, the Alexander teacher 'showed Mel where his posture was indeed misaligned'. 'Posture' is not a word in the AT lexicon. However, if you have back pain, go to an Alexander teacher and find out for yourself.

By now, and thanks to direct personal experience, I am well past the stage of 'I'll try it and see if it helps.' I am committed to the process that Alexander's principles imply. I continue with my weekly lessons – now with great pleasure – because it's like treating myself to dinner in a fantastic restaurant and at the same time learning to become a gourmet cook. And it's even much better!

After writing my original text, last year my teacher and I started to work on encouraging more cervical curve in my 'too straight' neck (which was already an improvement on the reverse curve I'd started out with).

During this work, I made the personal discovery that end-gaining is less effective than non-doing and thinking. To many this may sound obvious, but for me it constituted a real breakthrough.

Up until this moment, it had been very difficult for me to even recognise end-gaining in my Alexander work, although I had had no problem incorporating 'stopping' – inhibition – in my AT process.

I now perceive that this breakthrough occurred when 'Who cares if I slump or not?' became a watch-phrase. It's not, of course, that I wanted to slump ... or that I planned to slump ... but that I was finally not entirely oriented towards not slumping. This letting-go of my unconscious end-gaining of secretly and always wanting better posture re-oriented me to fuller attention on the means-whereby that Alexander offers us. This has curbed my end-gaining and enhanced the quality of my thinking and non-doing, both during lessons and in every-day life.

Every lesson now brings new benefits and new discoveries, thanks to my own doing less while thinking clearly. I have profited much from keeping this in mind, and now use it in conjunction with the idea of allowing flow instead of – however subtly – looking for some kind of better position.

When I was originally writing an account of my experience through having had lessons, I thanked the Alexander Technique for releasing me from my prison of pain. Today, I find I've stopped trying to fight the universe – and thank the AT for helping me cultivate flow in all aspects of my life.

# A Mindfulness Trail Through the Forest
Cherry Collins

I recently spent two weeks alone in the Scottish hills, in a cabin nestling in the shelter of the edge of a forest, looking down toward a beautiful loch. I am in my final year of Alexander Technique training to be a teacher, and my break in Scotland was an opportunity to reflect on what has brought me to where I am now in the Alexander world. I am also an ordained Buddhist, committed to a path of deepening mindfulness and spiritual growth in community with others. In addition, I have lived with a chronic health condition for many years now – ME (or chronic fatigue syndrome, as it is also known).

I have found the Alexander Technique the best way I can help myself develop increased health and stamina. I am so much stronger now than when I began my training. My Alexander story interweaves all these strands, and includes along the way my love of music, my experience of back and neck pain, and my own healing process through therapy with which the Alexander Technique helped and supported me. All our stories are individual – may aspects of mine speak to you in whatever form is helpful to you now.

My trail has been of long duration: starting a pathway, letting it peter out, finding another way at another time to pick up the trail. I have been hesitant, finding it hard to believe that the Alexander Technique could have the profound effect it has had on my health and wellbeing. I recognised in my first individual lessons it was something special that I didn't understand. It was something to come back to when I had changed, when time and circumstances were right.

So eventually, here I am on a training course. I never quite believed that the Alexander Technique, or Principle as it is sometimes called, could help with ME although I had a hunch that it would. This is how I come to be writing now. I would like to help make clear how this most baffling of conditions can be alleviated and helped by practising Alexander's discoveries. It is early days in my understanding, and I would be interested to be in touch with others who have explored this issue. I realise that the term ME describes a spectrum of symptoms, and it may be that my experience is unique. It has, however, become clear to me that the principles of the Alexander Technique can help anyone make the most of the condition that they live with – even if that is just 'life'. This applies vitally to people living with ME whether it is those with the condition or their carers. For us, energy is such a precious commodity which can be in very short supply.

The Alexander Technique teaches me how to channel my energy efficiently. It teaches me a mindfulness practice focused on the level of how our minds affect our reflex and muscular systems. It appears to be having the effect of 'waking up' neural systems in me that seemed to have shut down, or were struggling to be effective. I am learning to develop new pathways in my nervous system and this is having the effect of 'bringing my mind back' out of the cotton wool fog that can descend with ME. This mental fog has an ongoing debilitating effect, interfering with everyday activity and making it hard to hold down a job.

One of the toughest aspects of ME is its invisibility. Invisible illnesses are baffling for all. Learning the Alexander Technique as someone with ME is a very particular situation – engaging with a training course likewise. It is part of the healing process, and I have found out that it needs its own pace. When I try and rush or push my learning in any way I come a cropper! 'Direction' in Alexander terms is about the conducting of energy through the nervous system. In my experience it is addressing the very mechanisms in the body that have become faulty or broken down in some way.

One of the chief symptoms I experienced was a weakness in the neck area; it was as if all the strength had gone out of my neck and back. My head was so heavy. I needed chairs that included a neck rest, otherwise I fatigued very easily. I would prop my head up in ways I can now see probably exacerbated the problem. It was my experience that 'When there is weakness where the head and spine meet there is weakness everywhere'. This directly links into the heart of what the Alexander Technique teaches.

Our bodies are inherently unstable. We spend our lives responding to gravity, and that instability and flexibility are crucial to our wellbeing. The Alexander Technique teaches us to be aware of our whole body and mind, and how they work together. It trains us to use thought and direction of energy to influence how we approach any and every daily task. It uses the concept of inhibition to learn how to stop interfering in the way our bodies' efficient mechanisms work. It teaches 'direction' to enable us to choose positive patterns of thought so we interfere less with the smooth working of that mechanism. I have developed a greater subtlety of flexibility through my practice of the Alexander Technique as my body/mind system is gradually learning to work together more effectively. I am able to choose to develop more beneficial habits, literally lengthening in stature, widening in the torso and improving my breathing in the process.

The classic Alexander directions involve allowing the neck to free in order to send the head forward and up; letting the back and torso lengthen and widen; and releasing the knees forward over the toes and away from each other. If one is able to inhibit unhelpful tightening, retracting of the head and shortening in the body, one then develops flexibility and freedom throughout the whole musculoskeletal system. We gradually come to allow ourselves to operate in dynamic instability and freedom of movement.

At the heart of this system is something which F.M. Alexander called 'the primary control of the working of all the mechanisms of the human organism' usually shortened to 'primary control' in Alexander terminology. Alexander was discovering for himself in relation to his own body what eminent scientists of his day were exploring in relation to animals and the evolutionary development of humanity. Each of us can carry on that exploration in our own lives. The way that the head, neck and back work together is crucial to the functioning of the whole body system. We can observe in animals we see every day – dogs, cats, birds, and horses – that the head leads and the body follows. This applies to every animal that has a spine.

We stand upright on two feet, so it is easy to lose the connection – but it is still there! These days I am intrigued by the concept of primary control and use my everyday life as a laboratory in which to explore how it works, although when I first came across the Technique I found the term confusing and off-putting. Thinking it through more deeply, and gradually developing my own awareness of myself and the primary control operating within me, has led me to appreciate more fully its significance. This is especially clear when working with fellow students on the training course doing 'hands-on' work with them.

Walking the Scottish hills this summer I decided to experiment. Is the key area for the body's coordination really the neck/head/back relationship? As a Buddhist practitioner, I have spent much time gradually developing an awareness of my feet. It is something we learn to do as we deepen awareness of our bodies and the space we make in the world. I have noticed with myself and in looking around and observing others – especially in walking meditation – that awareness of the feet can sometimes lead one to draw oneself down in front, to 'pull down' in Alexander terminology. An understanding of how primary control operates can greatly enhance mindfulness practice.

Walking on steep hills, I noticed that my feet can lead, and they do so fine. If I forget my head, however, there is a heaviness in my step, and it's all a bit more hard work. My mind is watching, watching my feet. So I choose to 'let my feet go', moving automatically, and bring my main awareness to my neck and head, particularly where they meet at the base of the skull. Wishing for tension to undo. Allowing the anxiety of tripping on steep, rough ground to ease away. Asking – sending – my head up and away from that releasing neck, allowing my shoulder blades, my breastbone and collar bone to ease out as the muscles of my torso expand with the freeing breath. My hips too – tightness ungripping – and my legs coming out of my hips easily, lightly, swinging out from the torso. They know how far to step – they know how to move – and my spine releases up more as my feet touch lightly but assuredly on the ground.

My feet know where to go – they find the spot so long as my eyes are looking ahead, and a broad awareness fills my mind. I notice that there is less strain, it is less hard work. As someone with ME, my ability to walk used to be very limited indeed. At one time I used to need a stick if I went out, something I found hard as an ex-walker who loved the open air. My ability to walk has gone up, gradually.

I know, though, when I am 'flowing' walking and when the act of walking is a strain on my system. I could tell when I moved my awareness to the neck as primary focus, rather than the feet, that something changed. I also became aware of my feet in a new and more deeply connected way. My awareness of them came through muscular-skeletal connection; from inside, rather than an awareness from the 'outside-in'.

This is a snap-shot, an experiment conducted informally on my holiday. It has left me with a clear experience on which to reflect. Looking back on my own story of ME, it highlights for me that if the system breaks down around the area of the 'control centre' – the nape of the neck where the spine and skull meet – there are far reaching consequences. I used to prefer the term 'primary relationship' rather than primary control. As I have moved through my training course I have come to see that it really is the primary control.

It works as if it were a master code that we can all learn to use for greater ease, efficiency, health and wellbeing. For those of us with ME, it can mean the difference between accepting an invitation to a meeting or social activity or not. It becomes possible to trust that one's stamina will be available; that we have a method to enhance whatever stamina is available that day. It makes the difference between going for a walk, or feeling unable to make a step.

In Scotland, I have had a new experience for me of Alexander's 'directions', even 'orders' as he called them in the early days. As I pick my way up through the forest, finding sure footing, I hear Alexander's instructions for directing 'one after the other and all at the same time...' sound in my mind. They evoke what underlies the details of practical application. Intention. The key question. What is my intention?

Now, back home in an autumnal Sussex, I find a great time to explore primary control is when engaged in repetitive tasks which involve a lot of movement. I like exploring it while gardening: raking leaves, sawing with a pruning saw, planting spring bulbs. Doing these tasks can give us the experience of our back – the spine and the large muscles that dominate our back – being the powerhouse of the body. We can learn to allow that powerhouse to become more central in our awareness.

What is my intention? How is my neck now? Choosing to ask the neck not to grip around the task; choosing with that not-tightened neck to allow the spine to lengthen; sending the head, the crown, forward and up from our atlanto-occipital joint; allowing length between the tailbone and our 'nodding joint' between the ears. We can check as we move: am I expanding around this task or am I tightening, drawing in upon myself? How is the breath? Am I allowing it to move freely or has it tightened with my neck muscles and literally gripped the job too hard, stifling my life energy in the process?

I am at the beginning again of another journey. Each morning I start afresh with this learning. The task is to let go of my previous understanding and open to new discovery. These discoveries cannot be forced. They grow from observation and patience. I have learned so much on my training course – and I am very grateful to all my teachers who have helped me thus far.

## Round and Round the Garden: A Spiral Learning Journey
Carolyn Nicholls

When I had my first Alexander lesson, I caught a glimpse of something in my mind's eye. It was on the edge of my vision, a fleeting peripheral image of something wonderful. I didn't know what it was, it had something to do with my neck, and yet it seemed to be more than that. I decided I needed more lessons to find out what this glimpse was about.

There were days when, after my lessons, it felt as if my legs were carrying me of their own accord, that I wasn't actually walking – something else was 'walking'. It was strangely wonderful.

I had been nagged into having lessons by my mother who, suffering from ankylosing spondylitis, had received enormous benefit from her own lessons. She couldn't explain anything to me – although I would sometimes find her sitting in one of our dining chairs with her hands perched oddly on the top rail of another chair placed in front of her. It looked like she was playing buses, and I didn't understand. Finding her explanations inadequate, she booked me in for a series of thirty lessons. Those lessons changed my life, my career and my whole way of being. The Alexander Technique became a thread that ran through everything I did. My piano playing became easier, my damaged wrist, broken in an accident when I was twelve, grew stronger; I became calmer, taller, and suffered less pain. Up till then pain had been a fairly constant companion. I have a form of fibromyalgia, which meant I was often in pain when sitting or lying, or walking – or doing anything really. Climbing stairs would leave my thighs burning with pain after only two flights, sitting in a cinema was almost out of the question, as I would be in such pain at the end of the film.

I was having three lessons a week. After about twenty lessons I noticed my neck feeling different, and I could climb stairs more easily. I was intrigued. My teacher suggested I visit Lansdowne Road, where she

## The Primary Control of the Use of the Self

trained, and have a lesson with Walter Carrington. She had spoken about Walter quite a lot and I was curious to meet him, so I duly rang up, and was shocked at the length of time I'd have to wait for my lesson. Eventually, I climbed those mosaic marble steps to the big black double doors, rang the day bell and went in for my first lesson with Walter.

I remember this enormous hand sucking my neck up into itself like a limpet clinging to a rock, and there it stayed. Walter stood me, sat me, laughed, talked to me about rib cages. 'In our work, what we find is, people can tend to stiffen their ribs.' I nodded sagely. I knew that. He and I agreed on this point. It didn't occur to me until I was almost home that he was talking about my ribs, my stiffness. Surely not! I had had thirty lessons after all. I caught another glimpse, in the peripheral vision of my mind's eye – of a kind of freedom, an elusive but tantalising glimpse of a life free from pain. I wanted to see more, so I enrolled on the teacher-training course.

I thought I knew what it meant to free my neck, I was familiar with the directions: head forward and up, knees forward and away. But as I started training I felt I actually didn't know what they meant after all. It was a mystery; the glimpse of freedom left me, I felt mired in a morass of doing.

Later, I realised it was as if another layer of misuse was shedding – like a snake shedding its skin. My path became spiralic, mobius-like, a constant return to the much-loved and much-misunderstood (by me) concepts of inhibition and direction. It was like going back to the same piece of landscape year after year, walking round the same garden – seeing it again, fresh, new and yet familiar. The peripheral vision began to occupy centre stage in my sight lines and I could see more clearly the tools I was being given.

Training with Walter and Dilys was a privilege, and in those three years I formed lifelong friendships, gained another inch in height and acquired a reasonable pair of hands. Lessons with Walter were a highlight – his way of talking, which I came to call to myself 'the first person once removed' always intrigued me. He would engage you in a conversation about something – the neck, the knees, the thoracic area – and talk to you as if you and he were agreeing about the sorry state of such things – but you were equals and he knew that you knew about the neck, the knees, the thoracic area – he was just offering a gentle reminder. If you weren't paying attention, you could miss the delightful subtlety of Walter's discourses.

I qualified – another notch on the Alexander belt – and began to teach. The image of spirals stayed with me: a spiral staircase of use I climbed, occasionally looking back, sometimes seeing the same things from a different height. I began to write: lectures, articles, books. My learning felt almost alchemical in its subtleties and complexities. I pondered deeply on the effects of gravity on my neck muscles and wondered what the opposing force was, apart from my own muscles; perhaps it was the light itself, urging us upwards, like plants. From my new perspective of not only teaching the public, but also starting to be involved in training future teachers, F.M. appeared to be a magician.

I became Dilys Carrington's apprentice, learning the skills of teaching new trainees precisely what is involved in using hands on another person. Here, more than anywhere, I was struck by the seamlessness of use: how the things I had learned in my own early lessons were still the important things. How an understanding of good use was fundamental to becoming a good teacher and, if you wanted to teach someone else to become a teacher, you still had to maintain your own use.

'There, can you feel it coming?' Dilys would ask, her hand on the top of mine as we helped a new trainee into monkey. 'There it is, that's the direction coming.' I couldn't feel it – not at first. Later, I could feel it, even sense it coming before the sensation arrived in their backs, as she did. I could feel that Dilys was initiating this strong current of direction that began to flow through the trainees, and she was teaching them both to not interfere with its natural course and then to initiate it for themselves. It was all to do with the many facets of direction. 'Let's all let our knees go.' she would say; and we would, and the direction would flow from Dilys through me into the trainee, and on to the person they had their hands on. Everyone got it.

## The Primary Control of the Use of the Self

In 1987, the Alexander Technique took me to Australia – where it had all begun. I was the assistant on the first teacher-training course in Melbourne. Twenty-four people gathered from all over Australia for the course – some had never had lessons because at that time F.M.'s homeland had so few teachers. It felt strange and wonderful to be a part of re-energising Alexander's work in his own land, a strange spiral, an odd twist of fate. How would we fare? Peripheral vision now was fully focused on this way of working, this way of being and, to my pleasure, the more I taught and engaged others in the process of teaching, the more my own use improved. Long-standing injuries finally resolved and most of the time I was pain free.

Walter and Dilys came out to visit us in Melbourne, Dilys to see how her ideas were working out for me in our 'hands-on' sessions, Walter to lecture, discuss, give turns and share his thoughts. I was struck again by his immense skill and his beaming personality. He would work on our students, none of whom he had met before and somehow would find just the right way to talk to them so that things made sense. He talked to one about the rigging in a ship, how it had to be balanced if the sails were to catch the wind, how important it was that every rope was the right tension. He didn't know the man under his hands was not only a keen sailor but had built his own boat, including the sails! 'Must have smelt the salt behind my ears', was the astonished comment when the teacher moved on to the next trainee.

Sitting on the wooden veranda of our weatherboard house, waiting for the cool change to switch the air from stifling saturation to clean fresh breeze, was an opportunity for inhibition. I certainly couldn't change this stimulus – the cool change would come when it came – but I could change my response, so that I used myself better instead of fretting about what was not changeable. I learned a lot about use in different environments in Australia. Three years, a baby son and a flash flood later, I returned to the UK, glad to have lived for a while in F.M.'s homeland, to have visited Ballarat and Bendigo where he had taught, to get a sense of place and have seen for myself the 'wide brown' that must have influenced F.M.'s thinking. The sheer size and openness of the landscape, the immensity of the night skies and persistence of its people, these are now part of the Technique for me.

Of all the disciplines in my life, the Technique remains the one that is the most effective. Life throws challenges at you, both in the circumstances of your life and the accidents or illnesses that befall you. How you meet those changes is what makes you. I have been teaching over thirty years. My legs still sometimes hurt when I walk up stairs, but I don't make things worse by stiffening my neck or holding my breath as well, or shortening my spine.

Nor do I tell myself I'm not applying the Technique properly – an easy trap to fall into – 'Surely you should be perfect by now, shouldn't you!'

Instead, I return again to those things I was taught in my first lessons. How to free my neck, to send my head forward and up, to inhibit my responses so I can see my choices to act or refrain from acting more clearly. The glimpse I saw out of the corner of my eye is now a detailed picture, fully viewed. It is a landscape of body, mind, breath, awareness and choice that never fails to delight me. It is the journey I embarked on in my early twenties and I know will last me the rest of my life. Thank you F.M.

# Destiny Shapes Our Ends
## Ann Smith

Way back in the early 1940s 'good posture' as an item valued and encouraged by society first came to my notice – I would have been about fourteen. My straight-backed school friends were one by one awarded 'posture badges' at the end-of-term assemblies, watched enviously by me. So one term I tried really hard to put my shoulders back and stop slumping, to sit up, walk properly and all the rest of it, no doubt tensing all the more in the attempt. End of term arrived and found me ready to leap up and claim what I had surely earned – my posture badge. They were not impressed by my efforts and my name was not called. So I gave up, tried to forget it and pursue the more interesting things that were crowding around me.

In 1953, I was attracted to a small advertisement appearing in the New Statesman, the left wing weekly, for re-education. Something to do with posture and poise, and the re-education aspect put it well clear of failure and posture badges. Cheap, even free for deserving cases, it was sponsored by the wife of Sir Stafford Cripps, the Labour Chancellor of the Exchequer. They were both devotees of F.M. Alexander and felt that something so good should be available to anyone who wanted it.

I got myself and my son, a baby at the time, to Holland Park. My teacher sat me down and stood me up many times and then put me on a table and pulled my legs. It seemed strange but rather pleasant and she was unfazed by my posture and humpy, rounded back. She remarked that I was a rather tense person; tensely and meekly I agreed, seething within! At the end of the lesson I remember saying 'you make me feel like a princess', because what she had done was so good. But I was a little bit frightened of her and remarked, probably rather aggressively, that she reminded me of gym teachers. 'No,' she said tersely, 'I am an artist.' I was greatly surprised and felt I had put myself in the wrong, good and proper!

It was disappointing that my great adventure should end on this note. They offered me, I think, three free lessons which, regrettably, I never took up for various practical reasons. Maybe, too, there was a fear of taking the problem really seriously – and I felt I had gained so much in that one lesson in spite of my ambivalence about the teacher. Perhaps, in retrospect, it was as well, as the centre was run by someone who, I understand, had rather distanced himself from Alexander's pure method.

During the 1960s, Jungian analysis enabled me to change a great deal and discover more of who I was by working through some of the early-childhood emotional problems which were affecting my adult relationships – for instance with the Alexander Technique teacher. As therapy came to an end I set fair to 'de-stoop' and stand tall. But it seemed I could not: even then it took too much effort (of course, as I now realise) and, unable to keep up the impetus, determination dwindled. 'Trying' was a different kind of wrong way to express myself in all the movements of daily life, and just did not work. Meantime, I had changed my job from teaching young children to working with student teachers. Thirteen years later, I taught in schools again, at which point I really felt the strain of stooping and bending in the wrong places and my shoulders became more stressed, although I loved the work.

In the early 1980s and now living in South Buckinghamshire, I must have been ready for another encounter with the Alexander Technique – there is a destiny which shapes our ends!

Responding to an advertisement in the local press, I came to have lessons with a young teacher. She lived about five miles from my home and I think of her with affection. I remember her holding one of my legs off the table and asking in her gentle American accent, 'Are you going to give me your leg?' I think I had fortnightly lessons with her for about six months before she moved away to Cambridge.

She put me on to a friend of hers, a very good teacher she said, living in Aylesbury. So lessons continued. He was indeed, I thought, Alexandrian to the core and a very committed teacher. It was a long drive after school from Old Windsor but he would give me a cup of tea in his kitchen before lessons. He taught me that the Technique involves total coordination of the parts of the self, brain and nervous system, muscles, thought and emotions – the lot. Some of what he said, for instance about spirals, was hard to grasp and I felt constantly challenged. More than once he remarked that I was 'on beam' and I realised that all the transcendental meditation that my husband and I were practising, with its notion of 'doing less to accomplish more', probably helped.

He suggested that I might like to have the odd lesson with his own teacher in London. Again I did not take advantage of the offered opportunity – I certainly had no inkling of what I was missing and in any case I was very satisfied with his teaching. But alas, as he began to work more and more in London, in preparation for opening his own school in Aylesbury, he no longer gave lessons at home and put me on to another teacher who was, he assured me, very able and nearer to my home. I think I had been with the second teacher for about a year. The third knew what he was doing alright, but I did not feel in any way challenged, and knew I was not learning as much from him as from the first two. After a few months he too moved away and I did not seek out another teacher.

Why not? I was rather dispirited at that point and still, I think, felt the loss of the second teacher. I suppose I had a glimmering of 'leaving myself alone', but that dwindled as time went on. Not one of the teachers had stressed the importance of lying down in semi-supine position on a regular daily basis, so I did it less and less often. From time to time I thought the directions, but I had no notion at all of permanent primary control. I just did not realise that one needs to devote serious time and attention to the matter, that the Alexander Technique is a discipline.

Running a home, teaching full time, meditating regularly twice a day, gardening, going to art classes and concerts, socialising – I was busy, busy. So, gradually, I lapsed. At first I would sometimes rest in semi-supine during the lunch hour or after school, and even had the children doing it after movement lessons. But that was it; a little yoga and a lot of meditation constituted my self-improvement programme for the next quarter century or more. No more moves on the real re-education front from the early 1980s until 2006.

By now, widowed and settled into a different way of life, the prospect of reaching my eighties was only two years away, and I was beginning to feel 'past it', prematurely so I now realise. I was increasingly stiff, bent over, less and less able to straighten up, and very quickly tired: simple exercises from a do-it-yourself Pilates book seemed to cheer me up for a while, but they took so much effort. Old age was looming.

Then a few things happened which brought Alexander to my attention again. A couple of my friends remarked independently how much they were gaining from the Technique, one of them a good deal older than me. Then there was an article with photographs in the Guardian, about an Alexander teacher in St Andrews, in her nineties, still working and every morning doing yoga and walking the coastal path. Inspiring. Nearer to home a teacher in the next village advertised in the parish magazine – I'd often seen it – but, was she any good? A friend who had met her told me she was, at any rate, a very nice person and people spoke well of her work. Here, I felt, was a last chance, and within walking distance. I rang, liked her response and knew straight away that I was being handed something good on a plate. Now or never. This was IT. What luck!

She seemed to combine warmth, enthusiasm and concern, with just the right amount of rigour. In the kindest possible way she made it clear from the outset that to lie in semi-supine every day for about twenty minutes was more of a necessity than an optional extra, and produced an instruction sheet with illustrations. Pretty soon I got the message about the importance of inhibiting and directing as an all-day, lifelong commitment. But no chiding when, of course, I could not do it very much. She had been through all the problems herself, knew just where I was at and offered wonderfully firm yet light-hearted support – just what I needed.

After about sixteen months of weekly lessons I realised I had changed. I was slightly less crooked, more 'up', with greater mobility, energy and *joie de vivre* – almost young again. I could not have believed it possible, but it was happening. Every lesson was full of interest, and I read extensively and felt more and more drawn to the Technique. At my teacher's instigation I had the occasional treat of a lesson with her own teacher, in London. (No more passing up of great opportunities!) I attended a couple of courses, which broadened my experience of the Technique and made me want to learn more and more. Both my teacher and her teacher seemed to be offering me the option of doing some teacher training; no pressure, just a suggestion.

It was a big decision. I knew it would be taxing, especially at my age (seventy-nine) and that there would be neither time nor energy for much else. The journey would take at least an hour, incurring a change of trains – this in itself was tiring, especially on the way back after a morning of intensive work. But it was only for a term. Start in January and be finished by Easter, so I envisaged, as I decided to take the plunge. I had made preliminary visits and was wonderfully accepted and encouraged by the students. One youngish man said, 'the best thing I ever did', and a delightful American women in her sixties and near completion of the course made it clear that age was no barrier. It was irresistible, and on January 2nd, 2008 I began at the school.

After the first day I wrote, 'I am exceedingly tired. So much input from teachers. I experienced such lovely welcomes from teachers and students alike that I am thoroughly happy about it all.'

That first term was a revelation – so many 'turns', so many trained hands at work. At first I felt a complete novice, trying hard to do the right thing, but no one seemed to despair about me. It will come, was the message, direct up, will, wish and want, let the teacher do the work, use the eyes and so on. I was privileged to have the benefit of the co-head of training's care and expertise, but for only a little while as the cancer was advancing fast and he died on April 10th, having been absent for most of the term.

On 7th January I wrote that he was 'back, and he taught me about "monkey", very slowly and deliberately after he had had me standing, then sitting and standing once or twice. It seemed easier today or perhaps I am losing the need to "do it". He is so gentle and understanding. He stressed throughout "neck to be free", not to pull the head back and not to pull down in the front. I mentioned that I had realised over the weekend that my tummy muscles were tense. He said "think neck free, head forward and up first, and then tummy release, adding that the overall use is always more important than the little details – treat the whole and not the parts".'

His untimely death was a tremendous loss to the school, and the atmosphere was very sombre and sad as students and teachers alike mourned him.

Before the half term break, teachers were telling me that things were changing and I sensed it myself. Quoting again from my diary, one of the teachers 'got me standing in a way that seemed new. I said it did not feel like standing, it felt like something else. Why is all this so exciting and good? Because I think it is something I have never dreamt was possible, a true re-education, and at eighty!'

One of the students asked me what new things I had discovered in this first half term. I found it difficult to separate things out but later in my diary I wrote:

- I am much more 'up' and more aware of my back as a strong thing.
- Much more aware of ankles, knees, hips and indeed, legs in general.
- More aware of arms and their relationship, muscular, to the back muscles.
- 'Monkey' is no longer a complete muddle. I have had enough experience of a good 'monkey' to know how it can be.
- I have learned more of how the thought/wish/desire is what is needed, not 'doing' it. Head to tail as a unit.
- I am more in myself and can take more sensible decisions rather than be swayed by a desire.

By 28th February I had decided I definitely wanted to go on to a second term.

I often wondered what caused the difference between the two sides of my back: the right scapula was almost hidden in the stoop and my round shoulders, and the shoulders were at different levels. I am sure that my response to an almost perpetually tense atmosphere at home during my earliest years was to withdraw into a protective hunch. Also, I had an attack of pneumonia when I was eight. No antibiotics were available in those days and the illness caused a build up of pus around the affected lung that had to be removed surgically – an empyema. A drainage tube was inserted under the right shoulder blade, causing displacement which became a permanent feature of my anatomy – helped no doubt by my poor use, my hunch. A remark made to me by one of the teachers during this second term, and recorded in my diary, put the whole matter into perspective. She said, 'the aim is never to change shape but only(!) teach good use. One of my legs is shorter than the other and it's never going to grow.' In point of fact, a good deal of change of shape had taken place, but indirectly. As so often during my training, this was exactly what I needed to hear at the time, and it changed my attitude permanently.

During term two, the joy of learning about the soft placing of hands on the students in my group opened up another vista of the Technique – directing one's use not merely for one's own benefit, but for others. Of course I stayed for a third term, during which I wrote in my diary:

I seem to be taking the Technique into my everyday life much more often. To begin with, it's a novelty and one does it very occasionally. Then I started feeling guilty at how rarely I did it. I think it takes quite a while for the Alexander Technique to become really established in one's brain/mind/intention. I was feeling over the long weekend of snow etc. that the Alexander Technique is just undoing my lifelong way of going about living, and that only when having a lesson is one able to experience something else in its place. These last few days seem to have been an experience of 'Help!' I am stranded neither here nor there but almost suddenly today, I feel grounded again, with the Alexander Technique more firmly part of me.

During my fourth term (I had decided to stay on for as long as I could cope with it), I attended a weekend course and it was after this that I realised that I wanted to teach. So I completed nine terms, but because of increasing tiredness gradually cutting back to four days a week, then three, then two thus allowing plenty of recuperation time. This meant that I was short some sixty days, which takes a long time to accomplish at only two days a week! The school was moving temporarily and I could not face an even longer journey. To stop was a very painful but realistic decision and that is what counts. I can go in for the odd morning feeling totally welcomed by all and I exchange work on a regular basis. My home teacher, in the next village, and I work together every week, to my huge benefit. And I have a pupil! An old friend who is interested and knows I am not fully qualified, comes weekly for a lesson and this always energises me – no fee of course. So all is very far from lost. In fact, it feels just right.

Recently I have realised that if I let up on trying to inhibit and direct, my body does not like it and begins to hurt, proof that it appreciates better use, so one just has to go on living the Technique, willy-nilly! Apart from other benefits, it helps to keep me living in the present moment, neck free now, and maybe that is the beginning of wisdom.

Those nine terms working in close contact with younger students of many nationalities, taught by inspiring teachers, each with his or her own slant on the Technique, have constituted a wonderfully mind-broadening experience. Such a privilege at my age. I feel a never-ending love and gratitude toward them all for enabling me to experience the truth of Alexander's work, and for doing it with such humour, warmth and care. It was all such fun!

Now I am eighty-six, and old age has kicked in with its diminished energy and pains. I find balancing and walking rather problematic. But two things are tremendously helpful: daily Buddhist mindfulness meditation and practising the Alexander Technique with weekly lessons. *Awareness of body and mind.* I am fortunate to have had so much AT training whilst I was still able. Now it is simply essential for continued wellbeing.

I read somewhere that once, when F.M. was bidding an elderly pupil goodbye after her last lesson, he gave her this advice: to keep her neck free and to make sure she always had something to look forward to. Brilliant!

# Epilogue

Alexander Technique lessons turn out, as the stories in our collection show, to be an opportunity to discover that our preconceived ideas need revising. Initially, the AT lesson is an opportunity to experience what most of us know in theory, that 'what we think affects muscle tension and therefore also our posture', as Mary Rawson says. We have all come across the open, relaxed and balanced attitude of people who feel good, and whose wellbeing and confidence naturally induce them to 'walk tall'. Nor is it difficult to acknowledge the correspondence between worry, stress, depression, or anything we find difficult, and a tense, narrowed and pulled-down body.

What our authors are more astounded to discover through the simplest of acts – sitting and standing – is the excess muscular tension they bring to bear on seemingly banal and neutral everyday acts, and that this inappropriate pattern of response pervades a habitual psychophysical attitude toward life which largely predates the crisis or problem they are now wanting to fix – 'forty-five years of amassing a vast armoury of habitual responses culminating in a permanent back problem' in the case of David Green.

Alexander elaborated his method as a result of problems which he encountered as an actor – mainly hoarseness and voice loss – problems which, far from being triggered only by the overwhelmingly dramatic occasions of on-stage performance, also showed up in the way he used himself in normal, everyday speech. And if this non-dramatic build up of faulty use can end up having dramatic consequences after all, it is because its insidiousness prevents the problem from reaching consciousness. As Karen Scott-Barrett comments, 'I had not realised that I held extreme tension throughout my body all the time.'

Breaking down the action by suspending our automatic response to the stimulus not only gives us a chance to see what we are doing (to ourselves); it also gives us the space to unpack the different components of our psycho-physical habits and figure out what's what in the moment. Some storytellers, such as Anne Landa and Jane Evans, have been traumatised by sudden, shocking events, in these cases car accidents. Learning, from moment to moment, to say 'no' or 'stop' to the obsessive replay of the accident when awake – that is, to exert constructive conscious control over the memories of the incident – gives each of the authors a way of progressively disentangling and isolating the different strands which have been 'inextricably bundled' on a 'deep neuromuscular, physiological and psychological level'.

Without having to respond to quite so overwhelming a stimulus, most of our narrators acknowledge the fact that 'our physical self is bound to suffer if we are continually engaging in negative mental and emotional misuse' as David Green's teacher says. And if they tend to praise inhibition as an invaluable tool, this is precisely because being stuck in a perpetual cycle of negative thinking or unhelpful thought processes, even when there is no identifiable trigger or when the initial cause has disappeared, is one of the most prevalent among our bad habits. Many of the authors comment on this, directly or indirectly, including Christine Green, Mary Rawson and Janette Griffin.

A number of narrators express their sadness or regret at not being able to turn back the clock and discover the Alexander Technique at a younger age. But, as Alison Franks is quick to retort, 'you can never beat yourself up about what you didn't know. You can only beat yourself up about knowing something different and still not doing it'. The prevailing impulse running through the stories is to celebrate what the Alexander Technique enables them to do *now* that they could not otherwise have done – being 'an active hands-on Grandma' for Melody Hirst; going 'forward and up at seventy-five' by learning to walk correctly at last, for the sixth time, for Roey Burden; 'noticing a general feeling of youthfulness' for Peter Ribeaux; 'still making progress

*Epilogue*

at seventy-three' for the anonymous author of The Beagler; or simply 'getting the best possible use out of my body' for Thomas Newton.

Jane Evans recalls that before having AT lessons, 'I was beginning to think I was past my "best-before"', but concludes that 'now I knew that "the best is yet to be"'. This optimistic and forward-looking attitude echoes the advice which Alexander himself is supposed to have imparted to an elderly pupil after her last lesson: 'to keep her neck free and to make sure she always had something to look forward to'.

'Brilliant!', as Ann Smith, who reports Alexander's words, comments. The advice is 'brilliant' in its simplicity, whether or not the story itself is true, and in the self-evident link it establishes between being able to turn one's head freely (difficult to do with a stiff neck!) and choosing a constructive direction for one's life, regardless of biological time – a constructive direction that matches our deepest needs, one of which is surely to remain connected to oneself and to the world, so that in reaching out for others from a more effortless and balanced place we may also bridge the gap between who we wish to be and who we are. In the words of David Green:

> *I think we need to nurture this inner feeling of wanting to progress as a whole person. Perhaps it's a bit similar to yearning for a long-lost friend; but in our case our real self is not lost for ever; he's just around the corner and when we do meet up it's handshakes and smiles all round! ... To become a truly wholesome person is surely the way forward for everyone.*

*Claire de Obaldia*

# Glossary

| | |
|---|---|
| Ankylosing spondylitis | A chronic condition with a strong genetic predisposition in which the spine and other areas of the body become inflamed. It mainly affects joints in the spine and the sacroiliac joint. In severe cases, it can eventually cause complete fusion and rigidity of the spine. |
| Apnoea | During apnoea, there is no movement of the muscles of inhalation, that is, the individual stops breathing. Most common while sleeping. |
| Brachial plexus lesion | Brachial plexus injuries, or lesions, can occur as a result of shoulder trauma, tumours, or inflammation. |
| Charcot-Marie-Tooth disorder | A genetically and clinically heterogeneous group of inherited disorders of the peripheral nervous system characterised by progressive loss of muscle tissue and touch sensation across various parts of the body. |
| CT scan | X-ray computed tomography (X-ray CT) is a technology that uses computer-processed X-rays to produce tomographic images (virtual 'slices') of specific areas of the scanned object, allowing an internal view without surgery. |
| Diaphragmatic breathing | Abdominal breathing, belly-breathing or deep breathing is breathing that is done by contracting the diaphragm, a muscle located horizontally between the chest cavity and stomach cavity. Air enters the lungs and the belly expands during this type of breathing. This deep breathing is marked by expansion of the abdomen rather than the chest when breathing. |
| Diplopia or double vision | The simultaneous perception of two images of a single object that may be displaced horizontally, vertically, diagonally or rotationally in relation to each other. Normally, both eyes are still functional but they cannot converge to target the desired object. |

| | |
|---|---|
| Empyema | An accumulation of pus in the pleural cavity that can develop when bacteria invade the pleural space, often in the context of a pneumonia. |
| Fibromyalgia | Fibromyalgia syndrome is characterised by chronic, widespread pain and a heightened and painful response to pressure. Fibromyalgia symptoms are not restricted to pain. Other symptoms include debilitating fatigue, sleep disturbance, and joint stiffness. Some people also report difficulty with swallowing, bowel and bladder abnormalities, numbness and tingling, and cognitive dysfunction. Fibromyalgia is frequently associated with psychiatric conditions such as depression and anxiety and stress-related disorders. |
| Juvenile rheumatoid arthritis, also known as Still's disease or juvenile idiopathic arthritis | An autoimmune, non-infective, inflammatory joint disease of more than three months duration in children less than 16 years of age. |
| Meconium | A dark green liquid normally passed by the newborn baby, containing mucus, bile and epithelial cells. |
| MRI | A medical imaging technique used in radiology to investigate the anatomy and physiology of the body in both health and disease. |
| Multiple epiphyseal dysplasia (MED) | A rare genetic disorder which affects the growing ends of bones. |

*Glossary*

| | |
|---|---|
| Multiple sclerosis (MS) | An inflammatory disease in which the insulating covers of nerve cells in the brain and spinal cord are damaged. This damage disrupts the ability of parts of the nervous system to communicate, resulting in a wide range of symptoms, including physical, mental, and sometimes psychiatric problems. MS takes several forms, with new symptoms either occurring in isolated attacks (relapsing forms) or building up over time (progressive forms). Between attacks, symptoms may disappear completely; however, permanent neurological problems often occur, especially as the disease advances. |
| Myalgic encephalomyelitis (ME) | The common name for a group of significantly debilitating medical conditions characterised by persistent fatigue and other specific symptoms that lasts for a minimum of six months in adults (and three months in children or adolescents). The fatigue is not due to exertion, not significantly relieved by rest, and is not caused by other medical conditions. |
| Osteoarthritis | A group of mechanical abnormalities involving degradation of joints. Symptoms may include joint pain, tenderness, stiffness and locking. |
| Osteochondritis dissecans (OCD) | A joint disorder in which cracks form in the cartilage and the underlying bone, caused by blood deprivation in the bone. While OCD may affect any joint, the knee tends to be the most commonly affected. |
| Osteogenesis imperfecta | Sometimes known as brittle bone disease, it is a congenital bone disorder characterised by brittle bones that are prone to fracture. |
| Osteopenia | A condition in which bone mineral density is lower than normal. |
| Osteoporosis | A progressive bone disease that is characterised by a decrease in bone mass and density which can lead to an increased risk of fracture. |

| | |
|---|---|
| Paget's disease | A chronic disorder that can result in enlarged and misshapen bones. Paget's is caused by the excessive breakdown and formation of bone, followed by disorganised bone remodelling. This causes affected bone to weaken, resulting in pain, misshapen bones, fractures and arthritis in the joints near the affected bones. |
| Parkinson's disease | A degenerative disorder of the central nervous system. Early in the course of the disease, the most obvious symptoms are movement-related; these include shaking, rigidity, slowness of movement and difficulty with walking and gait. |
| Postural thoracic kyphosis | In the young, it can be called 'slouching' and is reversible by correcting muscular imbalances. In the old, it may be a case of hyperkyphosis and called 'dowager's hump'. |
| Prolapsed disc | Spinal disc herniation (in Latin *prolapsus disci intervertebralis*), commonly called a slipped or prolapsed disc. It is a medical condition affecting the spine in which a tear in the outer, fibrous ring of an intervertebral disc allows the soft, central portion to bulge out beyond the damaged outer rings. |
| Sacroiliac joints | The joint in the bony pelvis joined by strong ligaments. In humans, the sacrum supports the spine and is supported in turn by an ilium on each side. The joint is a strong, weight bearing joint with irregular elevations and depressions that produce interlocking of the two bones. The human body has two sacroiliac joints, one on the left and one on the right, that often match each other, but are highly variable from person to person. |
| Sciatica | Sciatica is a relatively common form of lower back and leg pain, but the true meaning of the term is often misunderstood. Sciatica is a set of symptoms rather than a diagnosis for what is irritating the root of the nerve to cause the pain. |

| | |
|---|---|
| Spondylolisthesis | A condition, either congenital or due to accident, in which a vertebra slips far forward of where it should lie due to fracture or malformation of the posterior processes. |
| Symphysis pubis dysfunction (SPD) | Separation of the two halves of the pubic bone at the midline. |
| Synovectomy | Removal of the synovial tissue from the knee. The principal role of synovial fluid is to reduce friction between the articular cartilage of synovial joints during movement. The synovial membrane seals synovial fluid from the surrounding tissue (effectively stopping the joints from being squeezed dry when subject to impact. |
| Trigeminal nerve | A nerve responsible for sensation in the face and motor functions such as biting and chewing. |

# Bibliography

Alexander, Frederick Matthias. (1995) *Articles and Lectures*. Mouritz.

Alexander, Frederick Matthias. (1997) *Constructive Conscious Control of the Individual*. Mouritz.

Alexander, Frederick Matthias. (1996) *Man's Supreme Inheritance*. Mouritz.

Alexander, Frederick Matthias. (2000) *The Universal Constant in Living*. Mouritz.

Alexander, Frederick Matthias. (1932) *The Use of the Self*. Methuen. Republished by Orion Press, 1985.

Alexander, Frederick Matthias. (1946) *The Use of the Self*. Chaterson.

Atkinson, Carla. 'Forward and Up at Fifty', *Conscious Control*. Vol. 2, No. 1, 2008, p. 20–30.

Barlow, Wilfrid. (1973) *The Alexander Principle*. London: Gollancz.

Campbell, Thomas. (2006) *The China Study: The Most Comprehensive Study of Nutrition Ever Conducted and the Startling Implications for Diet, Weight Loss, and Long-term Health*. BenBella Books.

Chesterton, G. K. (1908) 'Orthodoxy', *The Eternal Revolution*. Reprinted by Everyman's Library, 2011.

Desikachar. (1999) *Heart of Yoga: Developing Personal Practice*. Inner Traditions Bear and Company.

Dewey, John. (1932) 'Introduction', *The Use of the Self* by F.M. Alexander. Republished by Orion, 2001.

Eliot, T.S. (1943) 'Quartet 4: Little Gidding' in *Four Quartets*. Faber & Faber.

Goodman, Allegra. (2010) *The Cookbook Collector*. New York: Dial Press, Random House.

Hein, Piet. (2008) *Collected Grooks*, 2nd Ed, 4th Printing. Borgen.

Jones, Frank Pierce. (1997) *Freedom to Change*. Mouritz. First published as *Body Awareness in Action*, New York: Schoken Books, 1976.

Juhan, Deane. (2003) *Job's Body*. Station Hill Press.

Lewis, C.S. (1956) *The Last Battle: The Narnia Chronicles, Book 7*. London: The Bodley Head. Reprinted by HarperCollinsChildren'sBooks, 2009.

Macdonald, Patrick. (1989) *The Alexander Technique as I See It*. Brighton: Rahula Books. Reprinted 2002.

Morgan, Louise. (1954) *Inside Yourself: A New Way to Health Based On the Alexander Technique*. Foreword by Aldous Huxley. First published by Hutchinson & Co, UK. Reprinted by Mouritz, 2010.

Park, Glen. (Book, 2000; CD, 2005) *The Art of Changing: Exploring the Alexander Technique and Its Relationship with the Human Energy Body*. Ashgrove Publishing.

Shealy, C. Norman. (1999) *The Complete Illustrated Encyclopaedia of Alternative Healing Therapies*. Element Books Ltd.

Wolf, Jessica (2013) *The Art of Breathing*. http://www.jessicawolfartofbreathing.com/

# THE FM ALEXANDER TRUST

The F. Matthias Alexander Trust is a registered charity, which was established in 1991 in order to bring awareness and understanding of the Alexander Technique to the general public and to promote research and study into all aspects of the Technique.

The Trust is affiliated to the Society of Teachers of the Alexander Technique (STAT).

For information about the projects that have been supported by the Trust and how to apply for funding from the Trust please see the website. Proposals for projects must fulfill one or more of the aims of the Trust.

To continue the valuable and important work of the Trust, you can help in a variety of ways, for example, by volunteering to help or by making a one off or regular donations. You may also like to consider supporting the Alexander Trust in the long term by leaving a legacy in your Will.

The F. Matthias Alexander Trust
c/o STAT, Grove Business Centre Unit 48
560-568 High Road,
Tottenham, London N17 9TA

www.alexandertrust.org.uk